FINDING
YOUR WAY

FINDING YOUR WAY

A Medical Ethics Handbook
for Patients and Families

Katrina A. Bramstedt, Ph.D.

with Albert R. Jonsen, Ph.D.

Hilton Publishing Company • Munster, Indiana

Hilton Publishing Company
1630 45th Street
Suite 103
Munster, IN 46321
219-922-4868
www.hiltonpub.com

ISBN 978-0-9841447-3-0

Notice: The information in this book is true and complete to the best of the authors' and publisher's knowledge. This book is intended only as an information reference and should not replace, countermand, or conflict with the advice given to readers by their physicians or any ethicists. The authors and publisher disclaim all liability in connection with the specific personal use of any and all information provided in this book.

Grant E. Mabie, Managing Editor
Lynn Bell and Angela Vennemann, Editorial Assistance
Debby Dutton, Cover Design
Angela Vennemann, Layout and Interior Design

Publisher's Cataloging-in-Publication
(Provided by Quality Books, Inc.)

Library of Congress Cataloging-in-Publication Data
Bramstedt, Katrina A.
    Finding your way: through the maze of medical ethics in modern health care / Katrina A. Bramstedt with Albert R. Jonsen.
    p. cm.
    ISBN 978-0-9841447-3-0 (pbk.)
1. Medical ethics--Popular works. I. Jonsen, Albert R.. II. Title.
R724.B685 2011
174.2--dc23

              2011018556

Printed and bound in the United States of America
11 12 13 14 15 8 7 6 5 4 3 2 1

CONTENTS

Introduction

"Bioethics" and "medical ethics" are becoming everyday topics of stories in the media and even popular literature. We hope to reach the common reader, persons who might pick up and browse our book, rather than scholars. These lay readers are, we hope, healthy persons, but our book might help them think about these serious matters so that, in the event they, or someone close to them, become seriously ill, they will make better decisions when the occasion arises. Those occasions will be the moments when serious decisions have to be made about one's own medical care, or the care of a friend or relative. These decisions are needed amid the maze of ethical dilemmas that can exist. Many times, things are not clear at first sight, and complex questions are posed at a time when decisions must be urgently made. Emerging from the maze can only happen by examining deep ideas that most people don't think much about. These are the ideas of bioethics and medical ethics.

During the first decade of the 21st century, debates over stem cell research and the drama of Terri Schiavo, among other stories, captured wide attention. But laypersons, encountering these stories, are often baffled by the terms, concepts, and arguments that appear in them. Yet few persons need to understand them better, until they become patients themselves or when members of their family are hospitalized. A medical crisis is bad enough; but an unexpected ethical problem may cause deeper dismay. In the medical setting, the combination of stress, fear, complex technology, and time pressures can make medical decision-making difficult for patients and families. When troubling questions of ethics are mixed into this setting, distress and confusion abound. In this book we aim to unlock important concepts in medical ethics in order to aid patients and families in both health care planning and medical decision-making. Each chapter presents one topic that might arise in life, along with a fictional case setting the stage for discussion. The book also includes a list of helpful resources (Appendix A) and a glossary of frequently used terms in medical ethics and health care (Appendix B). We encourage readers to engage in candid discussions with their doctors about the topics and guidance in our book.

1

The Basics of Ethical Decision-Making

Consider the following scenario: *You and your sister are responsible for your mother's care in a nursing home. She is 81 years old and relatively healthy, but affected by rather serious dementia. One day, the nursing home calls to tell you that she has had a major stroke and has been taken to the local hospital. You rush over and meet the doctor in the intensive care unit. He tells you that your mother's condition is quite serious. She will not die, he says, but may have suffered major brain damage. When your sister arrives, the two of you, the intensive care doctor, and your mother's primary care doctor discuss the appropriate course of action. There is general agreement that aggressive treatment should not be applied and that a "do not resuscitate" order would be appropriate. You call your brother, a lawyer in the Midwest. He is angry that he had not been consulted about these decisions, says that he totally disagrees, and that he will be flying in tonight. The ICU doctor says, "Perhaps we should request an ethics consultation." Neither you nor your sister has any idea what that means.*

Put simply, an ethics consultation is a consultation about ethics. But "ethics" is not a very clear term. Webster's Dictionary defines the word as "motivation based on ideas of right and wrong." It's those "ideas of right and wrong" that confuse: different people have quite different ideas; different scholars provide different theories. U.S. Congressmen argue about an "Ethics Committee" that would monitor their conflicts of interest. The storms of war raise questions about the ethics of warfare, and the fears of terrorism challenge any such ethic. Preachers decry the lack of ethics in modern life, usually referring to dishonesty and sexual laxity. Despite killings and other crimes that most people find unacceptable, the Mafia are said to have "an ethic of loyalty." Physicians, lawyers, and accountants are held to the tenets of "professional ethics." K–12 educators wonder whether "ethics" can be taught; while college professors lecture on ethical theory. Often one hears, "Well, after all, everyone has his own ethics."

Ethics has long been a part of medicine. Doctors, from ancient times, have heard the advice of the Father of Medicine, the Greek physician Hippocrates, who said, "When treating a patient, be of benefit and do no harm!" This sounds simple and straightforward. But the reason we have "ethical problems" in health care is that it is often not clear what is a "benefit" is for a particular patient or how to achieve benefits without running great risks of harm. In most encounters between a sick person and a doctor, decisions are dictated by the patient's medical problem. For example, a worker, injured in a fall, has lost a lot of blood. As soon as the patient arrives in the Emergency Room, the doctor will immediately order a blood transfusion. Suppose, though, that the worker's wife arrives and says that he is a Jehovah's Witness and that it is against their faith to accept a blood transfusion. What should the doctor do? Honor their religious beliefs and let her husband die? Administer a blood transfusion in order to save his life and wait until he can confirm his belief later? Phone a local judge for an injunction? What is the right or wrong action for the doctors, for the patient's wife, for members of Jehovah's Witnesses, for the judge? This is one example of an ethical dilemma in medicine. How should we—or they—go about reaching that decision? This is a moment when someone might suggest an ethics consultation.

It might be said that this is a religious problem rather than an ethical one. The Jehovah's Witness belief is sincerely embraced by persons of that faith. It is based, they say, on certain words of the Bible. But when that belief is asserted in the medical setting, it becomes an ethical problem for all the health care providers. These doctors and nurses are bound by an obligation to benefit their patient and to avoid harm. They do not share the patient's religious beliefs. They strongly feel that failure to transfuse blood would harm the patient. They are unclear whether they have an ethical duty to respect a belief they do not share when facing a violation of their ethical duty to benefit the patient. Unquestionably, many ethical problems are based in religious beliefs, but most often in medicine, ethical problems may be based on more general ideas of moral obligation.

Although ethical problems have always been part of medical practice, they have expanded widely as many technologies for diagnosis and treatment have been added to medical practice. The modern physician has drugs, treatments, and machines that former physicians could not imagine. While it would seem that these additions would bring nothing but benefit, they almost always have negative aspects as well. In the most striking example, the machines that can support breathing (ventilators) can continue to do so after consciousness has been lost without hope of recovery. Is continued life in such circumstances a benefit or harm? What is the quality of life for a patient in this situation?

An almost reverse example is posed by the medical ability to save lives that are, in the eyes of some, deficient. Should very small, premature babies be saved from almost certain death, when they have the possibility of future difficulties in growth and learning? Should persons with severe limitations in mental development receive life-saving treatment? Should a convicted murderer receive a liver transplant? Bioethics has generally strongly supported treatment of such persons. The defense of a decision to withdraw or withhold treatment, or of a decision to provide it, requires strong reasoning and persuasive arguments. Bioethics is the specialty that is devoted to the careful, analytic study of such arguments.

Bioethicists generally agree that arguments about who should live, who should die, and who should decide must be based on several major ethical principles. The first of these is Respect for Persons. This means that every human being must be seen as a valuable and dignified participant in the human race. It also implies that each person should have the right to choose how they wish to live and how they will permit others to treat them. In medical care, this implies that treatments should, in ordinary circumstances, require the consent of the patient. The second and third major principles are Beneficence and Nonmaleficence (excuse the fancy terms, inherited from Latin). These principles, by definition, honor the teaching of Hippocrates, "Be of benefit and do no harm." They direct the doctor to focus his or her intentions on the welfare of the patient, not on profit or reputation. They acknowledge that almost every form of medical treatment involves risk, and require doctors, and their patients, to balance these carefully before choosing. The final major principle is Justice, the fair distribution of burdens and benefits within a population. This principle deals with broad social issues, such as health insurance, and with the policies for distributing scarce medical resources, such as organs for transplantation.

These four major principles provide general guidance, but they remain very wide and vague. Medical care is not about generalities but about very particular persons who seek help in illness from particular doctors who must apply their scientific knowledge and skills to this unique case. Similarly, bioethical problems must descend from the generalities of principles to the particulars of practice. This is the work of the mysterious "ethics consultation" mentioned in our opening case. A person trained in bioethics (an "ethics consultant") will usually begin by clarifying the particular details of the case that is presented. Many bioethicists will do this by summing up the circumstances under four headings that represent the common features of every medical case. The first of these four headings is Medical Indications: the facts and opinions about the patient's illness, treatment options, and expectations of success. The second is Patient Preferences: information about what the patient wishes regarding treatment or, if the patient is incapable of expressing wishes (that is, is unconscious or an infant), what choices, made by reasonable, impartial, and compassionate others, they might express or that would be in their best interests. The third is Quality of Life: an estimation of what the patient's life is likely to be, with or without treatment—that is, independent, mobile, pain free, capable of communication, etc. Finally, Contextual Features takes into account facts, not about the patient, but about the setting in which care takes place—for example, religious beliefs, financial circumstances, legal restrictions, etc. A bioethicist constructs a picture of the case by evaluating all these circumstance in the light of the four major principles. He or she is helped in this task of evaluation by a familiarity with the extensive writings about such problems that today makes up the literature of bioethics.

Evaluating the facts and principles as they appear in a particular case is the bioethicist's most difficult task. It is this difficulty that gives rise to the "ethics consultation." This is discussed in greater detail in the next chapter. A bioethicist may be a highly educated philosopher, but he or she cannot properly evaluate a case by reading books in the privacy of his or her study. It is necessary to bring together the participants in the case and to hear their views and their feelings. It is useful to propose for their consideration various options and the reasoning behind them. The aim is to move together toward a resolution of the problem that is reasonable, compassionate, and acceptable to all, or at least most, of the persons involved in the case. The following chapters offer brief examples of how a bioethicist might proceed in particular kinds of cases.

Let us return to our case. After your brother arrives, he spends an hour sitting at your mother's bedside. The next day, the ethics consultation convenes. Your mother's long-time primary care doctor explains the situation, and the neurology consultant confirms that damage from the stroke is probably quite extensive. The clinical ethicist explains that, in cases like this, in which prospects for recovery to health and consciousness are very dim, it is considered ethically acceptable to limit or discontinue life support. Your brother asks some lawyerly questions, then engages you, his sisters, in a serious conversation about what your mother would want in such circumstances. At the conclusion of that conversation, he says to you, "Well, I'm ready, if you are, to let Mom go in peace."

This ethics consultation has gone well; it provided information and allowed sentiments to be expressed. It led to a conclusion that each participant in the consultation judged reasonable and compassionate. More problematic cases are discussed in each chapter of this book.

KEY POINTS

- *Ethics involves moral choice—that is, applying personal and social values to the circumstances of particular events in order to determine the right course of action.*

- *Bioethics involves four social values of particular importance in medical care: respect for persons, beneficence, non-maleficence, and justice.*

- *In medical ethics consultation, the circumstances of particular cases are arranged under four topics: medical indications for treatment, the preferences of the patient, estimation of quality of life, and the influence of features of the context of the case.*

- *In order to resolve an ethical dilemma it is important to clearly understand the clinical facts of the case, as well as the patient's personal values about life and health care.*

2

HOSPITAL ETHICS COMMITTEES AND CLINICAL ETHICISTS

D r. Stephens, a cardiologist, is in a quandary. His patient, Mrs. Greene, is 82 years old and in the hospital's intensive care unit. She is being treated for her third bout of pneumonia in the past six months. She also has irreversible kidney failure requiring dialysis three times per week. Additionally, she has developed liver cancer, but she is not a candidate for a liver transplant due to her kidney failure and overall frailty. This frailty also prevents her from receiving other forms of treatment or surgery for the cancer. Dr. Stephens has asked for an ethics consultation about the ethical appropriateness of allowing the patient's pacemaker battery to not be replaced when it depletes itself. Dr. Stephens believes this would allow the patient to have an uninterrupted, comfortable death.

This is a very typical case for an ethics consultation. Ethics consultations are formal requests to help solve an ethical dilemma involving medical care. These consultations are in addition to other consultations performed by specialists to clarify particular problems that arise in the care of the patient. For example, Dr. Stephens may ask a kidney specialist to provide an opinion on Mrs. Greene's kidney function. For an ethics consultation, the hospital ethics committee or a clinical ethicist (should one be available) is called. An ethics consultation can be helpful in many different situations. For example, patients, family, or clinicians want to explore the ethical issues in a specific clinical case; the medical team is at an ethical crossroads with the patient or family and cannot find resolution; members of the medical team have strong and differing ethical positions about a patient's treatment plan; or a patient has no family or friends to help make complex medical decisions and the medical team cannot ascertain what the patient's values are.

Commonly, ethics consultations are called when the following ethical issues arise: a patient or patient's family is demanding forms of medical treatment that are non-beneficial (see Chapter 6); a patient is experiencing suffering that is difficult to control and a cure has yet to be found (see Chapter 7); a patient is refusing medical treatment that is life-saving (see Chapter 9); a patient is dying but the patient's family wants all life-support machines to continue (see Chapter 10); a child needs medical care but the parents are refusing such care (Chapter 15). Consultations can occur both for patients who are hospitalized and those who are outpatients.

Ethics consultations are handled by either an ethics committee or a professional bioethicist (also known as a clinical ethicist). In the United States, all hospitals, as required by the international hospital accreditation board (Joint Commission on Accreditation of Healthcare Organizations), have a mechanism to resolve ethical conflict. Most commonly, this "mechanism" is an ethics committee. The ethics committee is a group of people from a variety of disciplines, usually consisting of physicians, social workers, nurses, clergy, and one or more community representatives. It is desirable that these persons have some training in medical ethics. Training is provided within the institution or in short courses offered in many locales. These people respond as needed to requests received from patients, families, and medical personnel. Ethics committees usually have other duties as well, such as development of hospital policies about medical ethics matters, including the rules governing the process of deciding when and how to withdraw treatment from terminally ill patients. A clinical ethicist has advanced education in fields relevant to medical ethics (usually a doctorate in philosophy, theology, or social sciences) and practical training in clinical situations. Many large hospitals and academic medical centers employ at least one clinical ethicist, as their medical cases and ethical dilemmas can be more complex than those seen at small, community hospitals.

What should you expect if you request an ethics consultation? Usually, the clinical ethicist or a designated ethics committee member will review the patient's medical chart and interview the patient, family, physicians and nurses. Often these interviews are done separately, followed by a group meeting of all parties, if appropriate. It is important that all parties express their views and concerns freely. Using the principles of ethical decision-making described in Chapter 1, ethics advice will be given in written form to whomever requested the consultation. Usually, a formal consultation report is placed in the patient's medical chart, just as is done for any other specialty performing a consult (e.g., cardiology). The advice given in the ethics consult is just that—advice. Medical teams and patients do not have to follow the suggestions noted in the ethics consultation, but generally they respect and appreciate most or all of the advice given. It may clarify the terms of the dilemma that they face or bring reconciliation among family members. If a patient or family member is not satisfied with the ethics consultation advice, they have various options. They may appeal the recommendations to hospital authorities (an administrator or ombudsman). They may dismiss the doctor(s) with whom they disagree and seek another doctor. They may transfer the patient out of the hospital to another institution or, possibly, take the patient home.

In the case described, Mrs. Greene has what is called, in medical jargon, "multiple organ failure"—that is, several of her vital organs have ceased to function. Not only does she have permanent kidney failure but she also has terminal liver failure. There is no cure for these two conditions. She also has a serious heart problem, and the pacemaker is a form of life support. It keeps her heart beating at a rate fast enough to provide good blood flow to her brain. The fact that she is experiencing multiple bouts of pneumonia is of great concern: each time she gets sick, she is placed in the intensive care unit and requires breathing support with a ventilator. In other words, Mrs. Greene is a very sick lady.

The bioethics approach to this case would be to talk to the patient and explain the situation to her, suggest that these forms of aggressive treatment are merely postponing the inevitable, and ask her for permission to allow the pacemaker battery to deplete without replacing it with a new battery, explaining the consequences of this action (the beating of her heart would slow and then eventually stop). In this case, Mrs. Greene is making the decision in her own behalf, thus exercising her autonomy. Her providers may, and should, respect this choice. If the patient is too ill to make her own medical decisions and she does not have family or an advance directive that describes her health care values, the ethicist can offer guidance to the medical team. In this case, the guidance would be in accordance with the principles of beneficence and non-maleficence: what course of action would do the most good and avoid harm?

In the situation described, the common opinion of bioethics would maintain that it is ethically permissible to allow the pacemaker battery to deplete and not be replaced so that this terminally ill patient could pass away comfortably. This is because the patient has an underlying disease that is gradually leading to death and is causing her to suffer. Continued use of the pacemaker with a new battery only prolongs her suffering and postpones her inevitable death. (If the patient is well enough to make her own medical decisions, she can request to have the battery replaced, but some cardiologists might view this as futile and refuse to replace the battery. This ethical problem is discussed in Chapter 6).

KEY POINTS

- *Request an ethics consultation if you feel you need ethical advice.*

- *All hospitals have an ethics committee, and some also have clinical ethicists on staff.*

- *A clinical ethicist is a person with advanced education (usually a doctorate) and training in medical ethics.*

- *A formal ethics consultation report is generated for each consult. The advice given is only guidance for you and the doctors, not a requirement that must be implemented.*

3

THE SETTINGS OF
HEALTH CARE
ETHICAL DILEMMAS

Health care takes place in many different settings: the doctor's office, emergency department, intensive care unit (ICU), obstetrical suite, and on the general wards of the hospital. Patients are cared for at home or in skilled nursing and long-term care facilities. Caring for the sick, in any setting, can give rise to ethical problems, but certain settings are more prone to ethical problems. In this chapter, we look into some of the places where bioethicists find particular ethical problems and where they often are requested to deal with ethical problems. We will look into the doctor's office, the emergency department, the ICU, and the patient's home. Whatever the setting, patients and families should know that they are never alone in their distress and they always maintain access to ethics consultation, whether through a hospital ethicist, hospital ethics committee, or an independent ethics consultant from the local community.

THE DOCTOR'S OFFICE

You have been feeling unwell for several weeks. You have pain in your abdomen, some changes in bowel habits, and a slight fever. It will go away, you say, but your wife insists that you see the doctor. Finally, you call your primary care physician. The receptionist says that the next available appointment is in two weeks. When you say, at your wife's insistence, that you would like to see him sooner, she says the doctor can fit you in late this afternoon. You arrive and wait for almost an hour. When your doctor, a genial and competent fellow, sees you, he asks you to describe your symptoms, does a quick physical exam, tells you that you probably have diverticulitis, suggests a liquid diet for several days, then a low-fiber diet, and writes a prescription for an antibiotic. He also tells you that you should have a colonoscopy. And off you go.

Medical ethics starts the moment you need a doctor. Since the earliest times, physicians have been bound by the Hippocratic Oath: "I will use treatment to help the sick according to my ability and judgment and never to do them harm or injustice." The medical profession is built around the public trust that doctors will act always with the good of their patients foremost in their minds. Medical societies produce codes of ethics that spell out the various duties that their members have toward patients. The Principles of Medical Ethics of the American Medical Association open with the words, "A physician must be dedicated to providing competent medical service with compassion and respect for human dignity." The demanding principles of medical ethics, supported by strong social conventions and legal sanctions, allow anyone in need of care to seek help with confidence. Doubtless, there are physicians who fail to observe the duties—some are less than competent, some are without compassion and respect—but the average patient approaching the average doctor, even one totally unknown, can do so confidently.

The most familiar place for health care activities is the doctor's office or clinic in which the patient consults a physician. The physician may be one's personal doctor, called a primary care physician (PCP), or a consultant in a particular specialty, such as cardiology or dermatology. Also, nurse practitioners and physician's assistants work in these settings. Persons may select a personal physician (usually recommended by friends or found in the Yellow Pages). Some persons are members of health plans in which a physician from the plan is assigned to their care. The principal ethical problem in this setting is the very basis for ethics in health care: establishing and maintaining a therapeutic relationship between doctor and patient.

A therapeutic relationship means that the doctor acts with empathy, concern, and honesty toward each patient, treating each as an individual of worth and dignity, and that the patient feels that he or she can trust the physician, be confident that the doctor is dedicated to the patient's well-being, and be assured of his or her skills. Unfortunately, it is not easy for prospective patients to assess the medical competence of doctors. "Smarts" alone are not enough to create a good relationship between a doctor and patient. Consider an experience you may have had in the past with "bad service" when your doctor did not seem to listen to you during a three-minute exam. Even if you had time to explain your concerns, did your doctor listen? Is your doctor looking out for your best interests? Is your doctor deeply entwined with conflicts of interest (e.g., personal wealth or relationships with pharmaceutical companies) that might put your welfare secondary?

Be up front with your health care providers as to your needs and expectations. If you want a doctor who gives long visits and sits with you, and you value that as "therapeutic" in the relationship, then search for that. If you feel you have received service that is ethically inappropriate (e.g., the doctor was under the influence of drugs or alcohol, the doctor gave you a diagnosis without taking a thorough history or doing a physical exam, or the doctor crossed personal boundaries with you), you can report such serious breaches to the state medical board. Often, the local professional medical society will have a complaint review process as well.

Some matters are more nuisances than true ethical problems—for example, doctors who are late for their appointments or who fail to notify their patients when they are out of the office and appointments were planned for the day. True ethical problems are often avoided by honest communication between the doctor and patient on a consistent basis rather than waiting for problems to arise. One of the best examples of this is the need for patients and their PCP to discuss advance health care planning (Advance Directives, see Chapter 4). The PCP should be the first point of contact for these discussions about end-of-life care because the PCP, amid a therapeutic relationship, should be able to have a compassionate discussion about life, health, death, and treatment values with the patient. You, the patient, should feel comfortable having such a discussion amid this therapeutic relationship. After all, as death approaches, it is hoped that you and your PCP will be together, walking the final steps of life.

EMERGENCY ROOM

You and a friend are driving through an intersection when a big truck fails to stop at the red light and smashes into your car. The emergency room (sometimes called the ER or ED, emergency department) can be a scary place for patients and families. It is often very noisy, people are sometimes running or screaming, and paramedics are constantly arriving with more sick and injured to attend to. Sometimes, patients have heart attacks or seizures that are witnessed by other patients and families. Another cause of stress is the not uncommon waiting that occurs—for both patients and families, as the ER personnel usually cannot address all those in need when they arrive. Busy emergency rooms have a "triage" nurse responsible for sorting out those most in need of immediate attention. The sickest are seen first, and the others must wait their turn.

The physicians and nurses in ERs are extremely efficient and very busy. There is usually no established relationship between the care providers and the patients, unless the patients are "frequent fliers"—frequent visitors to the ER. Usually, little is known about the patient's medical history, unless there is a computerized medical record system that can help the medical team review any prior hospitalization records the patient may have. When there is no established relationship, the patient is an unknown; the team must diligently listen to the patient and family and address the symptoms to obtain a diagnosis and care plan. What often complicates these tasks is the fast pace of the ER setting. If a person arrives very sick and the team has no past history of the patient (and it cannot be provided by patient or family), the medical team has no understanding of the patient's health care values. In general, ER personnel assume that the patient wants treatment (that is why they came to the ER), but it might be that the patient did not (or they want limited forms of treatment).

While many patients get the care they need in the ER and are quickly discharged home, some require admission to the hospital for further treatment. Sometimes, in life-threatening situations such as severe organ disease or infection, admission is to the hospital's Intensive Care Unit (ICU). For those who are less ill, they are admitted to general ward units such as Internal Medicine. In the ER, interventions such as medication, sutures ("stitches"), and casting often occur in an effort to stabilize patients. Sometimes, patients require active assistance with breathing or blood detoxification due to kidney failure. These are interventions provided in the ICU. Sometimes patients refuse these interventions, and this causes the ER staff much concern; the reasons for these refusals needs to be explored very quickly (See Chapter 9).

INTENSIVE CARE UNIT

As with the ER, the ICU can be a frightening place for patients and families. The patient is very sick, sometimes close to death. The family is deeply anxious. The ICU itself is the ultimate in medical "high tech"; it is filled with numerous medical machines that often have many lights, alarms, and long pieces of tubing (often with a needle at the end). The patients in an ICU can be attached to many types of machinery at one time, each serving one particular organ or body system. For example, there are machines for feeding, breathing (ventilator), heart support (defibrillator, ventricular assist device, balloon pump), and kidney support (dialysis machine). Also, there are powerful medications that can keep patients sedated (asleep) for hours and days at a time so that they don't suffer as they undergo procedures and recover.

The doctors, nurses, and technicians who work in the ICU are highly skilled specialists. Patients seldom see their personal physicians (except perhaps as an occasional visitor) during their ICU stay. While ICU doctors and nurses provide care of the highest quality, they rarely come to know the patients very well—in part because they rotate frequently, due to the high intensity of the work. Patients and their families may get the impression that no one is in charge. They are unsure whom to question and, indeed, often get different answers from the many clinicians with whom they are in contact.

As subsequent chapters in this book will show, the potential of these machines and medications can be amazing, but they also set the stage for many ethical dilemmas. Often, the root of these dilemmas is the fact that patients in the ICU are critically ill and cannot communicate their health care values to the medical team. Also, they have not told their families about their values or written them down in an advance directive (see Chapter 4). When there is a plethora of technology to offer with a multitude of risks and benefits, decision-making can be difficult. Medical teams want to provide the care that the patient would want, but, in the absence of that, they sometimes have difficult choices to make on the patient's behalf. After a decision has been implemented, sometimes care plans need to be changed as the clinical status and prognosis changes. The critical nature of a patient's condition that brings them to the ICU sometimes leads to the tragedy of acknowledging that nothing further can be done to restore health or sustain life. The prospect of stopping life support (e.g., turning off a breathing or dialysis machine) or not performing cardio-pulmonary resuscitation (CPR) can be agonizing for family members (See Chapter 10).

HOME HEALTH CARE
Medical care in the home is often provided by family members, sometimes with the assistance of visiting nurses and physicians. Usually these patients are elderly and bed-bound, but sometimes they are children or others with a disabling illness that does not require full-time hospitalization. On-duty family members often wear multiple hats in that they are medical provider, spouse, parent, teacher, accountant, housekeeper, cook, and personal assistant. Sometimes their shifts last 24 hours a day, 7 days a week, with no breaks for national holidays or personal vacations (One useful book about caring for Alzheimer's

patients is called *The Forty-Eight Hour Day.*). The stress of these concurrent roles, combined with watching the loved one clinically decline (or fail to improve) can be emotionally overwhelming. Also, financial burdens can add additional strain.

A common ethical dilemma can occur in the home care setting. When the patient suffers a medical crisis in the home, it is almost instinctive to call 911 for emergency help. Even if a decision has been made while the patient was hospitalized not to resuscitate the patient, emergency responders will be ready to do their duty of resuscitating the patient and transferring them to the hospital. Overall, it is wise for the PCP, patient (if possible), and family to have a candid discussion about end-of-life care. The determination about cardiac resuscitation must be clearly understood by the PCP, the patient (if possible), and all family in the home (as well as all caretakers involved). Family members and home caretakers should be given clear instructions on what to do in such situations. Many patients do not want to die in a hospital or ambulance. To prevent this from occurring and to allow the patient to pass away peacefully at home, they should not be resuscitated by paramedics or transferred to a hospital for intensive care. These measures disrupt the patient's natural and expected death. In many states, laws allow for patients at home to have bracelets showing that their physician has ordered that resuscitation be omitted. The PCP can work with the family and a palliative-care or hospice program to help ensure that end-of-life suffering is minimized and death is as peaceful as possible (See Chapter 10).

KEY POINTS

- *Health care ethical dilemmas can occur in both inpatient and outpatient settings.*

- *Patients should establish a therapeutic relationship with their Primary Care Physician (PCP) and discuss their health care values with him or her.*

- *The Emergency Department is the setting for ethical problems arising from the fact that the patient is often unknown to the medical team.*

- *The Intensive Care Unit offers many medicines and technologies that can provide patients clinical benefit, but they also have the potential to create ethical dilemmas.*

- *Home health care can be a setting of ethical dilemmas, especially at the end of life.*

4

Advance Directives

S *cott, a computer engineer, was rushed to the hospital by ambulance when he collapsed at work. When his wife, Vivian, arrived at the hospital, she was informed that her husband had experienced a brain hemorrhage and was in the intensive care unit (ICU). The doctors in the ICU informed her that Scott's brain injury was significant. After a week, during which Scott had shown no improvement, doctors told Vivian that his brain injury was probably irreversible and that, if he did recover consciousness, it was most unlikely that he would ever gain meaningful neurological recovery. If he lived, he would never be able to communicate or make voluntary movements (e.g., walk, roll over, sit up). He would also need permanent assistance from a ventilator and a feeding tube. This information was emotionally devastating for Vivian, but she knew what Scott would tell her if he could communicate. Last year, Scott and Vivian each completed an advance directive that stated their wishes if they were to become terminally ill or suffer permanent unconsciousness. Vivian kept a copy of Scott's advance directive in her purse, and Scott kept a copy of Vivian's in his briefcase. Vivian showed the document to the medical team, and they read Scott's value statements about quality of life and "life on machines." Together, Vivian and the team agreed to withdraw life support within 72 hours, giving the rest of the family time to arrive and share Scott's final days together.*

An advance directive is also known as a living will. This document is a written statement made by an adult, describing one's values about medical care. In this document, a person tells family members and the medical team the extent to which he or she wants treatment when faced with a devastating prognosis such as a terminal illness or permanent unconsciousness. These documents can be prepared prior to any serious illness so that, if illness strikes and the patient cannot tell doctors what they want and don't want, some expression of their wishes are available. The advance directive communicates when the patient cannot—either because the patient does not have the physical means to communicate (e.g., talk, write) or because the brain is not working and the patient cannot mentally process information.

Advance directives typically contain sentences such as "If there is no reasonable expectation of my recovery from a seriously incapacitating or lethal illness, I do not wish to be kept alive by artificial means." Many states have passed laws that endorse these directives. These laws usually contain examples of acceptable documents. However, any adult may write a document expressing personal wishes (although it is advisable to get guidance from one's doctor).

An advance directive can be typed or handwritten. Also, advance directives do not have to be prepared by or signed by an attorney, but in some states they do need to be witnessed and/or notarized. No official form or format is required, but some people choose to use templates provided by various organizations. In the United States, each state has its own template, and these can be found at the following Web site: www. caringinfo.org/stateaddownload. Other templates (Jewish and Catholic directives) are listed in Appendix A.

An important part of the advance directive is the designation of a surrogate decision-maker. This surrogate, also known as the attorney for health care, is the adult person assigned to make medical decisions on behalf of the patient when the patient cannot make his or her own decisions (in this case, the term "attorney" does not mean that the person so assigned must be a lawyer). It is advisable that individuals designate a primary surrogate and also an alternate surrogate. This is because sometimes the primary surrogate cannot be located or is otherwise unable to function as decision-maker. It is not a good idea to appoint two parties as joint surrogates, because this can create unclear boundaries between the parties. Instead, it is highly advisable to assign primary and alternate status.

It is very important that you appoint someone who knows your values and is willing to honor them. As discussed in Chapter 1, the duty of the surrogate is to ensure that *your* values and treatment preferences are honored. This can sometimes be difficult for surrogates to do when these values differ strikingly from their own. Surrogates can be tempted (consciously or unconsciously) to project their own personal values when making medical decisions, so it is very important that they know your wishes and be willing to uphold them. It is also important to have a frank and clear discussion of your advance directive with your doctor and to be sure that he or she has a copy on file. This is because, when a patient is admitted to the hospital in an emergency, the patient's personal physician is usually notified and is sometimes the first person to become aware of the situation. It is important for your personal physician to know your values and wishes about health care. Words on a piece of paper can be helpful guidance, but, because they are always quite general and vague, the interpretation by someone you trust and who knows you well is very useful.

Additionally, you should review and revise your advance directive as your life situation changes. For example, if you get divorced, you may or may not want your former spouse, whom you had designated in your advance directive, to be your medical decision-maker. If one of your surrogates dies or you have a falling out, this too would change your options. If your health status changes and you become chronically or seriously ill, you may have more time and experience in the medical setting and certain events may have changed your values about the treatments you want and don't want. If, for instance, you receive a powered device such as a pacemaker or implantable defibrillator, there may come a time in which it should be turned off (so that you can die without suffering or prolongation of your illness).

In the case described, Scott and Vivian planned ahead and each prepared an advance directive. Vivian not only knew the values of her husband but also honored these values by supporting the treatment wishes he declared in the document. These wishes meant allowing her husband to die by withdrawing the life-support technology that had been started. Also, the medical team showed compassion to Vivian by allowing her family time to travel to the hospital so that they could spend time with Scott during his final hours of life. In this case, an ethics consultation was not needed, because the patient and his surrogate had anticipated the ethical dimensions of their futures and provided for them by a well-recognized technique, the advance directive.

Key Points

- *All adults who have the ability to make important decisions should complete an advance directive. No official form or format is required. The document can be typed or handwritten.*

- *Advance directives do not have to be prepared or signed by an attorney.*

- *Appoint a durable power of attorney for health care (a primary surrogate) and an alternate surrogate.*

- *Give a copy of your advance directive to your surrogates and your primary care physician and discuss your values with them.*

- *Review and revise your advance directive as your health status or values change.*

5

Do Not Resuscitate Orders and "Code Blue"

Jacob is 80 years old and lives in a nursing home. His two children visit him every weekend. They are very devoted to him and ensure he has the best of everything, including physical therapy, art therapy, and weekly massages. For the past week, Jacob has been in a hospital intensive care unit (ICU) due to pneumonia. He is on a ventilator and fed with a tube placed down his nose and into his stomach. He has also developed some heart beat irregularities that the doctors are trying to treat with medication. At times, his heart rate slows considerably. Jacob does not have an advance directive. The medical team has approached his family on several occasions and advised that, should Jacob's heart stop naturally, the technique called cardio-pulmonary resuscitation (CPR), which could restart his heart-beat, should not be performed so that Jacob could pass away peacefully. His family, however, are adamant that they want the team to "do everything" to save their father, including CPR.

"Do everything" is a common instruction to medical teams by families, even when "everything" includes medical procedures that are not helpful and are, in fact, harmful. Cardiopulmonary resuscitation or CPR is often included in the "do everything" request, despite the dismal success of this procedure for very sick patients. It is helpful for patients and families to understand what CPR is and what it can and cannot offer.

CPR is a technique used when the heart and lungs stop working. This is usually referred to as an "arrest." A person who has suffered an arrest is sometimes described by medical personnel as "found down." In the medical setting, this emergency is known as a "code blue" because a patient's skin often turns a bluish color when it is no longer getting an adequate supply of oxygenated blood (blood with oxygen in it). CPR is a procedure involving chest compressions (pressing down on the chest) and artificial respiration (inserting oxygen directly into the patient's mouth with a tube). The brain needs oxygen for health, and the source of this oxygen is its blood supply. The action of forcing oxygen into the patient's throat has the potential to send it into the lungs where it can dissolve into the blood and be carried to the brain. The action of pressing on the chest can physically move blood from the heart to the brain when the heart has stopped pumping. Getting the blood to move by physical force when the heart has stopped beating requires strong pressure on the chest, and this can sometimes cause a patient's ribs to break, especially if the patient is frail or elderly.

Often, powerful heart medicines (e.g., epinephrine, atropine sulfate) are given to the patient during CPR in an effort to assist the mechanical attempt to get blood to the brain. Also, sometimes the heart is given one or more electric shocks with a device called a defibrillator. A defibrillator is a small device that has a computer connected to two "paddles." These paddles are placed on the patient's chest and electricity travels from them into the patient in an attempt to restart a heart that has completely stopped (or to correct a defective heart rhythm). All these events happen very rapidly, because every second counts. The longer a person is "down" the risk of brain damage increases because the brain continues to be deprived of oxygen. This brain damage may be permanent.

These procedures can be life-saving. An otherwise healthy person who has a sudden heart attack and is quickly resuscitated by someone who knows how to do it can be snatched from instant death. Thus, many persons who have suffered an unexpected cardiac arrest while at home or at work are alive today because of rapid application of CPR. Also, persons who have had a surgical operation may experience heart difficulties during recovery; CPR will save their lives. However, in general, the success rate of CPR for hospitalized persons is very low. While medical professionals are aware of this, the general public is generally not. Television shows depict inevitable success. Visions of George Clooney successfully reviving patients in their hospital beds are often vivid in the minds of many family members. In reality, formal research studies have shown gloomy results for CPR, regardless of whether the underlying problem is a traumatic injury (gunshot, car crash) or disease. This is particularly so when the patient suffering a heart attack is also not a healthy person, but rather a person seriously ill and hospitalized. In a study conducted in an ICU in Germany, 169 patients received CPR between 1999 and 2003. Of these, only 80 patients survived and left the hospital (47.3%). Of these 80 patients, 12 (15.0%) were severely disabled and 2 (2.5%) remained unconscious.[*]

Because of these dismal results and the fact that CPR is not gentle on the body, physicians sometimes advise families that

---

[*] Enohumah, K. O., O. Moerer, C. Kirmse, J. Bahr, P. Neumann, and M. Quintel. 2006. Outcome of cardiopulmonary resuscitation in intensive care units in a university hospital. *Rescuscitation* 71(2): 161–70

CPR *not* be performed on patients who are in the process of dying from some underlying disease. CPR will only add to their suffering, and it will not reverse their clinical course. Even if CPR does interrupt death, it merely delays death in a dying patient. The patient will live to die another time, usually soon. Also, as shown by the results from the German study (and others), even when "successful," CPR can revive patients to a worse state than they were before they arrested—alive but permanently brain damaged. This is because, while a patient is "down," the brain is deprived of oxygen, causing brain cell death (brain damage). When CPR revives a patient, it does not cure any brain damage that occurred while the patient was "down." When it works, CPR only restores the heartbeat and lung function.

Even for those patients who are not actively dying, but who have multiple medical problems and a burdened quality of life (see Chapter 7), physicians sometimes advise that do not resuscitate (DNR) orders be considered. The reasons for this are the same as those stated above. Patients who are already significantly clinically burdened are very likely to have their burdens increase by experiencing a poor outcome with CPR (brain damage). Sometimes CPR is not even offered to patients because medical teams know in advance that it will not work (and only cause harm). In such cases, CPR is deemed futile or non-beneficial. This is discussed in detail in Chapter 6.

In the case at the beginning of the chapter, Jacob is 80 years old and appears to have lived a wonderful life with a caring family around him in his last years. The medical team fears that CPR would not succeed in restoring normal heart function or, if it did, the success would be brief and transitory. In the unlikely event that CPR did succeed, the patient might be permanently neurologically devastated, unable to communicate or even eat without the use of feeding tubes. Because Jacob does not have an advance directive and cannot communicate due to his illness and attachment to the breathing machine, the situation is very complex. In the setting of an ethics consultation, the ethicist would meet with the family to explain the low chances of success for CPR and the burdens even of success. The ethicist would ask the family to describe the values of the patient in an attempt to understand what his wishes would be if he could communicate them.

Knowing that Jacob is Jewish and that Jewish teaching is quite strict in the matter of withholding medical treatment, the ethicist asks the family if this is a consideration. They answer that the family is not particularly devout but that they have heard a sermon in which the rabbi stated that if a treatment did more harm than good, it could be omitted. The conversation then focuses on this point, and, on hearing the doctors and the ethicist explain the burdens of CPR and even of its "success," the family agrees that they have no duty to subject their father to these consequences. If the family had focused on the high failure rate and insisted that, even with such low chances, they wanted their father resuscitated, the issue of "futility" would come to the fore. This topic is discussed in Chapter 6. In the last analysis, however, the decision of whether or not to perform CPR is a medical decision that is made by the medical team. If the medical team determines that CPR has no medical utility—that is, if it will not work and will in fact cause harm—they have no legal or ethical obligation to perform it.

Key Points

- *CPR is a valuable life-saving method but only under rare, favorable circumstances.*

- *CPR is infrequently successful in the hospital setting, and, even when it "works," the outcome can be worse than before CPR occurred.*

- *CPR is physically traumatic and can result in broken ribs.*

- *CPR interrupts the natural dying process, and, for some patients, this interruption prolongs suffering.*

6

NON-BENEFICIAL MEDICAL INTERVENTIONS

G lenn's wife, Alice, is in the intensive care unit. She has cancer that has spread from her lungs to her liver, bones, and brain. The doctors have told Glenn that Alice likely has only a few days left, even with use of the ventilator, feeding tube, and dialysis. The doctors have suggested that these therapies be stopped so that Alice would die from her disease in a peaceful way. Alice has been in a coma for the last two weeks and has no advance directive. Glenn is demanding that the doctors start another round of chemotherapy, as well as use a special "herbal tonic" from Tahiti. In fact, a nurse saw Glenn attempting to pour the tonic into her feeding tube on one occasion. The doctors have told Glenn that Alice's cancer is very aggressive and has spread so much throughout her body that chemotherapy will not be effective. Also, they feel that Alice is too weak and frail for it. Because chemotherapy is highly unlikely to work and will very likely cause significant adverse effects, the doctors call it "futile"—that is, without benefit. They say they have no obligation to use non-beneficial treatments, and refuse to proceed. This *angers Glenn, and he has threatened to tell this story to the local television station and to bring legal action against the hospital.*

Science has given modern medicine many forms of treatment. When patients are dying or suffering, many therapies are tried, and many bring great benefit. Unfortunately, science has not found a cure for every disease or symptom, and, even when a treatment is known to be effective, it never works in *all* cases. These facts put patients, families, and physicians in difficult situations when cures that are highly improbable are demanded. Physicians have an ethical obligation to provide medical therapies only to patients who have the capacity to benefit from them. Sometimes doctors cannot predict with certainty who will benefit from a particular therapy, so the therapy is used on a trial basis to see if it will work. If it works and the side effects are tolerable, then the therapy is continued. If the therapy does not work it is stopped. Such treatments may be called futile (or non-beneficial) because they are very unlikely to produce the desired result.

Modern medicine depends on a scientific understanding of how the body works in health and disease, and of how various treatments affect health. Medical treatments are constantly studied for their effectiveness and safety. Physicians constantly read the results of these studies. In the case presented, they would find that the medical studies reveal that continued chemotherapy for advanced cancer such as Alice's is statistically demonstrated to be ineffective. They would also discover that there is no mention in any scientific literature of the Tahitian tonic. They also have their own personal experience with the success or failure of various methods of treatment. This does not necessarily exclude the rare possibility that some treatment might quite unexpectedly work, or that a patient may improve while receiving it, but doctors can only decide on appropriate treatment by scientific studies and their own experience.

In addition, many very effective forms of treatment cease to be useful because the patient's condition has deteriorated so badly, or because disease has become so extensive. In these cases, it is not so much science as experience that tells the doctor that further treatment is futile. Many doctors are reluctant to make such a crucial decision on their own; they will seek advice from informed colleagues. It is rare, then, that a judgment of futility is made without serious consideration.

"Futility" itself is not a scientific term. It may be supported by some scientific evidence, showing very low or no probability of success, but it cannot be definitively proven, because a future improbability may, by chance, turn probable. However, common sense judgments, bolstered by as much data and experience as a competent physician can muster, must be taken seriously. There are limits to every expenditure of human effort.

Futile treatments don't cure patients or relieve their suffering. They *can* harm patients, however, because they can cause side effects. For example, giving a patient a cycle of chemotherapy that is very unlikely to work puts them at risk of serious infection, nausea, vomiting, rashes, hair loss, and bone pain. Such treatments can also give patients and families false hope. Some clinicians might choose not even to offer them. Overall, there is no ethical or legal obligation to provide futile treatments to patients, even when they are vehemently demanded. Ethics and the law have traditionally honored the precept "ought implies can"—that is, no one can be obliged to do the impossible. Physicians cannot be ordered to provide futile treatments, and insurance companies, in general, won't pay for them if they are implemented when explicitly known to be non-beneficial.

In the case of Alice and Glenn, the medical team has determined that chemotherapy will not be beneficial to Alice due to her specific clinical situation: the spread of her cancer to vital organs. While this is upsetting to the patient's husband, the medical team should make an attempt to help him understand that they have her best interests in mind and that they do not want to harm her. It might be helpful for the medical team to show the radiology images to the patient's husband, explaining to him in detail the extent of the spread of the cancer. The doctors, or perhaps Glenn himself, might ask for an ethics consultation. It is certainly an ethical dilemma to determine whether a treatment benefits or harms a patient. If an ethicist was involved in this case, discussions about benefits and harms would be prominent, as well as reflections on Alice's personal values about health and life. Even if the spouse still refuses to allow withdrawal of life support, he should be encouraged to accept the terminal diagnosis and impending death so that he can spend quality time with his wife in her last hours of life.

KEY POINTS

- *Futile treatments do not cure patients or relieve their suffering.*

- *Futile treatments can harm patients.*

- *Futile treatments can give patients and families false hope.*

- *There is no ethical or legal obligation to provide futile treatments to patients.*

- *Physicians have an ethical obligation to be good stewards of medical resources, which means providing medical therapies only to patients who have the capacity to benefit from them.*

7

QUALITY OF LIFE AND TREATMENT BURDENS

William, age 19, lays in the intensive care unit with his parents keeping vigil at the bedside night and day. Six days ago, he was the victim of a head-on hit-and-run car collision that caused him to eject through the windshield of his truck. Since arriving at the hospital, he has been receiving full life-support measures, including a feeding tube, ventilator, dialysis, blood transfusions, and medications to elevate his blood pressure. His heart stopped once, and he was revived after 20 minutes of CPR. William's brain damage from the car crash and cardiac arrest was severe and probably will cause permanent defects in his ability to communicate and connect with his environment. He is now delirious, slipping in and out of consciousness. When conscious, he does not communicate understandably or recognize his family. The medical team has advised the family that William does feel pain and that he requires large doses of pain medication to control it. He also requires medication to control agitation. After several weeks, the medical team advised William's parents that life-support *interventions are keeping him alive, and he could likely live for some time more (possibly up to a year) in a nursing home if he received a tracheostomy (permanent breathing tube placed in the neck), continued dialysis three times per week, and a percutaneous endoscopic gastrostomy tube (PEG tube, a permanent feeding tube inserted through the stomach wall). Another option would be to withdraw life support, allowing their son to die. William's parents agonize over the situation. His mother cannot accept his loss; his father reminds her that William is a vigorous athlete, a collegiate state champion kayaker and avid mountain climber. He asks, "Would he want that kind of a life, even for a short while?" The doctors recommend an ethics consultation to aid them in their decision.*

The concept of "quality of life" is not easy to define. If you asked 50 people to define it, you likely would get 50 different replies. In the most general sense, quality of life refers to a life that is "healthy, wealthy, and wise." More realistically, it may refer to a life over which a person has some degree of control and which is relatively free from pain and suffering. This pain and suffering has physical, psychological (emotional), financial, and spiritual components. Diseases of all sorts impair quality of life, sometimes only temporarily and sometimes permanently. A severe cold can make life very unpleasant, but "we get over it." Various forms of cancer may cause severe pain and debility; these symptoms may be controlled or the cancer may go into remission. Diseases such as multiple sclerosis or Parkinson's effect irreversible damage on the body and on the independence of the person who suffers them. Yet humans are remarkably resilient. Even persons living with severe disease can master their suffering. For such persons, "quality of life" is impaired, yet they might tell us that they are satisfied with their lives.

Often, intensive medical treatment adds further distress to the suffering of the disease itself. The hospital setting certainly does not enhance quality of life. Even when hospitalization is temporary and the treatments ultimately successful, there are many inconveniences. In the hospital setting, even patients who are semi-conscious can experience agitation that requires medication or even restraints (arms tied to bed rails). Procedures such as insertion of needles, catheters, endotracheal tubes (for breathing), and even routine turning from side to side can cause pain. Feeding tubes placed down the nose and into the stomach are well known to cause irritation. Many medications have unavoidable side effects such as body pain, nausea, vomiting, dizziness, constipation, and anxiety. Procedures such as placement of a trachestomy tube for long-term breathing assistance come with the risk of infection. Similarly, patients who receive permanent feeding tubes because they cannot swallow or take food via mouth or for other reasons also risk infection. This is because, even though there is no food entering the stomach through the mouth, the mouth and airway area still have a supply of saliva that can be a choking hazard. When patients choke on this saliva, it can cause a condition called aspiration pneumonia, which requires use of antibiotics and, usually, a ventilator (sometimes temporary, sometimes permanent).

Every conscious and communicative person can express his or her own quality of life. People can say they are feeling fine or miserable. However, it is a difficult challenge to make such judgments about another who is unable to communicate. It might even be said that it is impossible to accurately describe the quality of life that someone else experiences. We can only witness the external portion of an individual—their visible expressions, actions, and words. We cannot feel (and thus truly know) the emotions and the physical pains that someone else is experiencing because we are not neurologically connected to them. This fact complicates medical decision-making by persons who must make decisions on behalf of others, called "surrogates." Almost always, surrogates find themselves representing patients who cannot express how they are experiencing their life, and cannot make choices about how they want to live. Yet complex medical choices must be made. Sometimes, these choices involve therapies that, if not started (or removed), will result in the death of the patient. Other treatments may continue to support life, but it may be a life that is profoundly diminished in quality. Surrogates have to ask themselves, *What would the patient want?* As discussed in Chapter 1, the duty of the surrogate is to facilitate medical decisions that are in keeping with the *values and wishes of the patient* (not the surrogate) if these values and wishes are known.

While intensive care physicians are generally well-skilled at identifying and treating symptoms that impact patient quality of life, sometimes difficult clinical cases emerge. Examples include trying to control a patient's severe agitation without using complete sedation, as well as control of intractable nausea. In these situations, a physician specializing in palliative medicine, the control of pain and suffering, should be consulted to offer guidance in managing the patient so as to optimize pain relief and eliminate or reduce symptoms. This is also discussed in Chapter 10.

Another matter to consider is the setting in which a person's life is experienced. In the ICU, quality of life can be impacted by many different forms of invasive medical technology. As has been described, some of the technologies cause pain and suffering, as well as agitation. Often, however, these patients recover and transition back to their prior state of health and quality of life. Those who are ill but not hospitalized may also have their quality of life severely impacted by their illness. Examples include patients who have severe disabilities yet live at home or in nursing homes, such as patients who have suffered strokes or who have debilitating diseases like multiple sclerosis or Lou Gehrig's disease (ALS or amyotrophic lateral sclerosis).

These people, while they usually do not require invasive medical procedures, often have lost much of their independence and rely on others for care and assistance. This lack of independence can be emotionally devastating for them. Also, the lack of physical activity can impair their quality of life.

For some people, quality of life is more important than quantity of life. Said another way, these people would rather live a life that is shorter but contains less pain and suffering than a longer life. Others value a life that is as lengthy as possible, no matter how much pain and suffering occurs along the way. When faced with the option to die naturally, instead of having life artificially prolonged with machines such as ventilators and dialysis, some people choose to continue aggressive treatment against the odds. Unless the medical team determines that such treatment would be futile, patients should have their wishes honored (See Chapter 6). A surrogate should reflect seriously on what he or she knows about the patient when making medical decisions on behalf of him or her.

In this case, William's surrogates, his parents, may recall his vitality and the life that he loved. They now know that, not only will he never return to this life, but that he will be burdened both by his physical condition and by the treatments required to keep him alive, and that this will be so as long as he lives. This may form the basis for a judgment about William's quality of life. An ethicist might guide them through the next steps: Do they believe that William himself would choose to live this diminished life? Do they believe that such a life is in his best interest? If they can suspend their own feelings and honestly answer yes to both questions, it is reasonable and compassionate to discontinue life support. Although some bioethicists maintain that life should be sustained regardless of its quality, such a decision, carefully and reflectively made, has general support within contemporary bioethics.

KEY POINTS

- *Many patients value quality of life over quantity of life.*

- *Quality of life includes both physical and psychological perceptions.*

- *Quality of life can be severely impacted by symptoms such as nausea, vomiting, pain, anxiety, shortness of breath, and loss of independence.*

- *A palliative medicine specialist should be consulted to assist in the treatment of severe symptoms that are difficult to manage.*

8

PATIENT PRIVACY AND CONFIDENTIALITY

S *ue is a patient in the cardiac intensive care unit, where she is recovering from heart bypass surgery. She is awake and alert and has provided a list of names of people that she does not want to visit her during her hospital stay so that she does not get overstressed while she is recovering. She does not want these people to even know that she is hospitalized. Sue's sister, Jane, who is mentioned on this list, repeatedly calls the hospital seeking information about her sister. Sue's husband tells Jane that Sue has been sick for the past few days, so Jane arrives at the hospital to try to find her. When the receptionist refuses to give her Sue's room number, she becomes angry and insists on seeing a hospital administrator. During an elevator ride, she watches two doctors view a chest X-ray by holding it up to the ceiling light. She sees her sister's name on the image and also hears them talk about her heart surgery.*

Privacy includes a person's right to exclude others from one's own physical, psychological, and informational space. Most people value their privacy. In the hospital, people lose some of their privacy: they may share a room with a stranger, be clothed in revealing hospital gowns, and be cared for by an almost anonymous crew of doctors and nurses who read their personal information in the medical chart. This crew shares that information, and their impressions, at every shift and staffing change. Confidentiality, the duty not to disclose private information to unauthorized parties, is a traditional duty of health care providers. Only persons responsible for the patient's care and treatment are considered authorized. Also, persons close to the patient, such as spouses, domestic partners, and family, have traditionally been considered authorized. However, today, with so many persons involved in care and so many means of communication, this obligation is under pressure. Also, in recent years, limits have been set even on family and friends who formerly were included in the circle of those with whom information can be shared.

Discussions between doctors and patients are private conversations, but physicians usually write or dictate notes that summarize the discussion and highlight significant points. This is important in order to provide the best care possible for the patient, as doctors cannot commit to memory everything they hear and must communicate with others responsible for care. There are times, such as emergencies, when these notes need to be quickly shared with others who are not directly affiliated with the patient or physician without the patient's permission. The most difficult situations involve information that pertains to the potential endangerment of other parties (including knowledge that a patient has a serious contagious disease such as hepatitis or tuberculosis, or that a patient is making threats to physically harm others). In the United States, all states have laws that set limits on information disclosure, but, frequently, the cases require complex assessment of what personal or social interests can justify a violation of privacy.

Often spouses and partners want to know the medical details of their partners' conditions. In the United States, privacy laws do not allow doctors to automatically disclose this information to the partner (or other legal next of kin) unless the patient has given permission for the doctor to do so. Occasionally patients may want to keep their diagnoses secret from their families. In these situations, doctors must keep the diagnoses private (unless they pose a safety hazard to others), even if a family demands to be informed. Exceptions to this include a patient who is incapacitated due to the illness and does not have the ability to provide such consent and treatment decisions need to be made. In this case, the doctor must inform the appropriate person who has authority to make these decisions.

Confidential medical care for minors is a complex issue. At times, young people who are not adults and are still living with their parents may seek medical attention for a condition that they do not want their parents to know about. According to the American Medical Association Code of Ethics, "Where the law does not require otherwise, physicians should permit a competent minor to consent to medical care and should not notify parents without the patient's consent." Parents can often be helpful to their children with regard to medical matters such as contraception, pregnancy-related care (including pregnancy testing, prenatal and postnatal care, and delivery services), treatment of sexually transmitted disease, drug and alcohol abuse, or mental illness; however, sometimes fear or shame may deter young people from seeking medical help. If a doctor feels that parental notification is justified in order to aid the child's treatment, he or she must discuss the reasons for the notification with the child *prior* to the disclosure. Notably, in the United States, some states have laws that require parental notification for certain types of treatment (for example, methadone for drug abuse treatment). There are also some state laws that prohibit parental notification without the minor's consent.

In an attempt to provide a minimum level of privacy in U.S. hospitals, a federal regulation known as HIPAA (Health Insurance Portability and Accountability Act) was enacted. This regulation was created to protect patients from unauthorized release of their personal health information. This means that there are restrictions on who can view the contents of a person's medical records and how this medical information is shared with others. This regulation also allows patients to see their own records and to designate persons who should be permitted or not permitted to visit them when they are hospitalized.

Confidentiality of medical information, then, is very strict. Still, there are situations in which some outside party claims to have the right to that information. Most significantly, public health authorities do have the right to know facts about a patient that might indicate that the person is a threat to the health of others. Also, criminal law enforcement has the right to know facts that are relevant to the commission of a crime. These exceptions are usually codified in law. Insurers have the right to know certain information supporting claims for payment, but usually this is disclosed to a patient prior to medical procedures.

In the United States, some have attempted to use a person's residency status as a method of rationing health care. There is not a system of universal health care in the United States, and patients are required to pay for their medical costs via their own personal insurance or personal funds unless they qualify for public assistance (for example, Medicaid). For those who are not U.S. residents, their immigration status often makes them ineligible for public health care insurance and hospitals sometimes fear their medical services will go unpaid. Nonetheless, it is unethical (and a violation of privacy) to inquire about a person's immigration status as a contingency to receive health care in the setting of a medical emergency. Medical care should be provided to anyone who needs emergency medical services without regard to their immigration status (or their ability to pay).

In the case described, Sue has the right to set limits on who she wants to allow to visit her in the hospital, and, according to federal regulations, these limits should be supported by the hospital team. Consultation reports, lab test results, and X-rays are forms of personal medical information. Often, doctors need to discuss these items as a team in order to share their medical knowledge and experience, yet patient records are private and should be discussed in private settings so that people not related to the case are not exposed to other people's personal information. Certainly, the elevator is not an appropriate place for doctors to talk to each other about their patients (unless no other people are in the elevator). Usually, doctors converse via private phone or meet in the patient's hospital room or in a conference room. Professionalism requires that doctors uphold the dignity of their patients in all their discussions. If Sue's sister had requested an ethics consult with regard to access issues, the ethicist would have explained the U.S. HIPAA regulation to her.

KEY POINTS

- *Among its many provisions, HIPAA protects patients from unauthorized release of their personal health information.*

- *Sometimes doctors release medical information about a patient to others without the permission of the patient.*

- *Professionalism requires that doctors uphold the dignity of their patients in all their discussions.*

9

Refusing Medical Treatment

B ob, age 40, is a patient on the endocrinology unit. Four
days ago, he drove himself to the hospital's emergency room
after feeling weak. The medical team discovered that Bob
had diabetes, as well as gout, and several open sores on his legs
that appeared to be infected. He was also dehydrated and ane-
mic, requiring a blood transfusion. Bob agreed to be admitted to
the hospital, but, after four days, Bob told the medical team he
wanted to leave. The medical team indicated he was still sick and
needed further hospital treatment. The nurse saw Bob looking for
his street clothes and personal belongings and informed the attending physician that Bob was seriously planning on leaving.

Hospitals can be very confining places that keep individuals
away from their friends, family, pets, and jobs for sometimes
extended periods. The well-known surroundings of their own
bed, kitchen pantry, and favorite clothes get replaced with a
hospital bed, hospital food, and a hospital gown. The treatments given often have unpleasant side effects, and the daily

regimens are often very rigid, with many rules that people do not have in their "normal" routine. These issues can sometimes create anxiety or tension that results in patients desiring to leave the hospital before their course of treatment is complete. Medical professionals term this behavior leaving the hospital "AMA" (against medical advice).

Leaving AMA is the most extreme example of refusing treatment. In other situations, patients decide to stay hospitalized but refuse certain treatments while there. For example, a patient might refuse to eat, take medication, or allow blood samples to be taken. A patient might refuse to allow the doctors to insert a catheter or breathing tube. The medical team takes these situations very seriously, because physicians have an ethical duty to find out why a patient is refusing things that are clinically needed. When the treatment offered is life-saving, and the refusal will result in the patient's death, the medical team must ensure that the patient has given an "informed refusal." An informed refusal must be honored: legally and ethically, persons have the right to accept or refuse medical treatment.

A patient cannot give an informed refusal unless he or she has decision-making capacity. When a patient has decision-making capacity it means he or she has the ability to receive information (written or verbal), understand it, think about how it applies to the clinical situation at hand, and then express a choice about what to do (accept or reject the proposed treatment/procedure). A person who is comatose, intoxicated, heavily sedated, or confused does *not* have decision-making capacity. Also, some clinical conditions impair the ability to make decisions. For example, people who have large amounts of carbon dioxide in their blood or high fevers often cannot think clearly. Persons who refuse treatment in this situation will be told that their refusal cannot be honored and must be given an explanation as to why. Similarly, incapacitated patients who are asking or attempting to leave the hospital AMA will be prevented from doing so. Sometimes this requires a sitter or security guard to be placed in the patient's room to ensure that he or she does not escape. There are legal procedures governing this sort of restriction, and they must be followed.

Patients who have decision-making capacity can make an informed choice to refuse therapy, even life-saving therapy such as dialysis, intubation, and CPR. Sometimes, a patient can change his or her mind and request that treatments previously consented to be stopped. In these situations, it is very important that the medical team verify that the patient has the mental capacity to make a clear, deliberate decision, especially if treatment cessation would result in death or deterioration. If decision-making capacity is verified, life support can be removed at the request of the patient. U.S. law has supported this drastic decision. Because death is permanent and irreversible, medical teams, however, want to be sure that patients understand this consequence when they, themselves, request withdrawal of support.

In general, children cannot refuse clinically needed treatment because they lack the capacity to make decisions of such consequences. This is discussed in detail in Chapter 15. Courts sometimes allow older children (teenagers) to refuse medical care if the judge believes that the child has the understanding and emotional maturity to make an informed refusal. These situations are reviewed very carefully by a variety of personnel, included physicians and psychologists, especially if the cases involve refusal of life-saving treatment such as chemotherapy or radiation and the chance of cure is high.

Perhaps the most commonly discussed cases of informed refusal involve Jehovah's Witness patients refusing blood transfusion because their church forbids such treatment. A similar example is that of Christian Scientists, who generally rely solely on prayer for healing and refuse most types of medical treatment, with the occasional exception of surgery. In these situations, religious values are at the root of the treatment refusal. To the non-believer, these values seem illogical, even "crazy"; however, for the patient who holds these values they are very important. When adult patients express these values, medical teams must honor their wishes, even if the consequences are as severe and permanent as death. In some cases, judges have allowed teenage Jehovah's Witnesses to refuse life-saving blood transfusions. Children, however, should usually be treated, regardless of their parents' denial of permission (see Chapter 15).

In the case example, it needs to be determined if Bob has the mental ability to make his own medical decisions. The ethics consultant can assess the patient to determine his ability to give an informed refusal and help educate him about the clinical need for the hospitalization. If it is determined that the patient has the ability to make an informed decision to refuse treatment, he should be allowed to leave the hospital even though the physicians do not feel it is medically in his best interest. If it is determined that Bob does not have the mental ability to make his own medical decisions, this means that he cannot make an informed choice to leave the hospital. This also means that the hospital can decide to take the legal steps to keep Bob in the hospital to receive medical treatment. In another scenario, doctors sometime determine that patients are so mentally unstable that they are a danger to themselves or others. In these situations, patients can be placed on a "mental health hold" (forcibly held in the hospital for evaluation and treatment until it is safe for their discharge). These latter cases are handled by psychiatrists and the legal system rather than ethics consultations.

Key Points

- *Adults with decision-making capacity can refuse any type of medical treatment, including life-saving medical interventions.*

- *Adults who lack decision-making capacity cannot give an informed refusal for medical treatment unless they have made prior statements to this effect (when they had capacity, for example, as part of an advance directive or verbal statements to family or health care providers).*

- *In general, children cannot refuse clinically needed treatment.*

- *Courts can order forced treatment (medical and psychological).*

10

HEALTH CARE AT THE END OF LIFE

M ary is 90 years old and has spent the past week in the intensive care unit (ICU), sedated, on a ventilator. She has a long history of lung problems that have required her to use an oxygen tank at her bedside at home each night. She has been living with her daughter and son-in-law for the last 15 years. Recently, she lost her desire to eat and told her doctors she did not want a feeding tube, even if it meant she would die without nutrition. She also did not want to be kept on a ventilator if she could never again breathe on her own. Because Mary required 24-hour sedation while on the ventilator, she could not speak to her family or the medical team. Knowing that Mary would not be able to live without full-time ventilator support, the medical team approached Mary's daughter to talk with her about end-of-life care. The team suggested that Mary be removed from the ventilator now, rather than wait another week, as it would not change her prognosis. It would also place further burdens on her to keep her in the ICU for therapies she would not want. Mary's *daughter was quite distressed by this suggestion and said she could not make such a decision—at least not right away. Mary's doctor proposed that an ethics consultation might aid her to think through her options.*

As discussed in Chapter 7, attempts to cure disease often require the use of procedures and therapies that cause pain or other side effects (e.g., anxiety, nausea, vomiting). At the end of life, when a patient is dying, this added suffering can be avoided by changing the goals of treatment. When the goal is to cure a disease or illness, many forms of aggressive therapy and procedures are often implemented. These can include ventilators, dialysis, blood transfusions, feeding tubes, chemotherapy, radiation, and surgery. Sometimes, despite the best efforts of the medical team, the progress of the illness cannot be slowed, or trying to cure it becomes too burdensome or risky for the patient. In these situations, it is medically and ethically appropriate to withdraw the treatments that are not working, as well as those that have become too burdensome (harmful) for the patient. Similarly, situations arise in which it is medically and ethically appropriate to not offer or provide certain treatments to patients for the same reasons: they either would not work or would cause excessive suffering.

These decisions to withdraw or withhold treatments are not arbitrary. Procedures, drugs, and other interventions are only withheld if it is felt that the patient would not benefit from them or if it is known that the patient would not want them. Doctors may write do not resuscitate (DNR) and do not escalate (DNE) orders in these situations. A DNR order tells other doctors and nurses who care for the patient not to restart a patient's heart once it has stopped. A DNE order directs the medical team to maintain the patient's current level of treatment but not to add additional aggressive interventions, other than increased pain relief (or other comfort measures) if necessary. Sometimes patients and families ask medical teams to "do everything" at the end of life, but "everything" often is not clinically appropriate. While the pharmacy may be stocked full of medication, there might be only one or two drugs that are suitable for each specific patient depending on the unique clinical situation. Similarly, the hospital may employ the best surgeons in town, but, if the patient is too sick to undergo surgery, the procedure itself could cause death if performed. The medical profession does have much to offer patients, but not everything it has to offer is appropriate for every patient. "Doing everything" does not mean that the patient should receive all the drugs in the pharmacy; it obviously means that the doctors should do everything that is clinically suitable for this patient at this time.

Some people confuse withholding and withdrawal of medical treatment as forms of euthanasia or physician-assisted suicide. When a medical procedure or drug is withheld or withdrawn from a dying patient, the patient's body continues in the dying process without being interrupted by the presence of that procedure or drug. In these situations the medical team does nothing to actively cause the patient's death; the patient dies as a result of whatever illness is present. Euthanasia, however, is the active killing of a patient, by someone other than the patient. This can be performed by anyone and by any deadly means. For instance, a husband places a plastic bag over the head of his wife. It can also be done by a doctor administering an overdose of drugs or poison. In situations of euthanasia, the patient's disease does not cause death but rather death is caused by the drug or poison. Euthanasia is considered murder in the United States and in most places in the world. Physician assisted suicide (PAS) is the act of a patient committing suicide using medication prescribed but not administered by a physician. As with euthanasia, the drug directly causes the patient's death, not the patient's underlying disease or illness.

Because suicide itself is not illegal, some jurisdictions—such as the Netherlands, Switzerland, Belgium, and the state of Oregon in the United States—have legislation that permits PAS under very strict circumstances.

When the goals of treatment are shifted from life-saving interventions to providing comfort to the patient during the process of dying, we speak of "comfort care" or "palliative care." Within a comfort care approach, invasive machines such as ventilators and dialysis are not used. Drugs designed to cure (e.g., chemotherapy) are also not used. The care plan becomes one in which control of pain and suffering is the main priority for the medical team. Often palliative medicine specialists are consulted so that the best care plan can be formulated. These specialists are experts in identifying and managing symptoms such as pain, agitation, nausea, vomiting, and shortness of breath. Often, these patients are managed as part of a hospice program. Hospice programs are set up in inpatient, outpatient, and even home settings where patients receive care that is designed for comfort, symptom control, and emotional support (of patient and family), while the underlying disease continues to advance, eventually causing death. These hospice programs are not limited to the elderly or those with cancer. There are special hospice programs for children. Hospice services generally include a team of people such as doctors, nurses, clergy, social workers, and therapists who assist the patient and the family as the patient transitions to death. Hospice programs also assist the family for a period of time after the patient has died.

In Mary's case, the ethics consultation determined that there was a clear medical consensus that Mary was terminally ill— that is, in the active process of dying. In a family meeting, that consensus was fully explained to Mary's daughter. The burdens that continued curative and supportive treatment would impose on Mary, without hope of any reversal of her dying, was extensively and sympathetically discussed. When Mary's daughter was invited to reflect on her mother's values as a person, and her wishes regarding medical care, she realized that the most compassionate course was to refrain from further life-sustaining technologies and treatments. As a result of this discussion, Mary's daughter, with the support of her husband, decided to allow her to die in a peaceful, hospice setting. While death of a loved one is emotionally devastating, knowing that the patient's values were honored at the end of life can be an emotional benefit to those left behind. Removing the ventilator allowed Mary to be moved out of the ICU and into a quiet hospice unit, where there were no machines, alarms, or painful procedures. The focus of Mary's hospital stay switched from curing her disease to alleviating her symptoms and allowing her to have a peaceful death.

Key Points

- *At the end of life, the goals of medicine shift from curing disease to alleviating symptoms and comforting the patient.*

- *Withdrawal of life-support technologies is a form of comfort care that allows the patient's disease to progress, uninterrupted, to death.*

- *Withdrawal of life-support technologies is not euthanasia or physician-assisted suicide.*

- *Palliative medicine specialists create detailed care plans that focus on controlling burdensome symptoms such as nausea, vomiting, anxiety, insomnia, pain, and shortness of breath, as well as the emotional and psychological distress that accompanies dying.*

- *Hospice is a setting in which the patient experiences a comfort care approach at the end of life and death is expected within six months.*

11

TRANSPLANT ETHICS

B arbara has end-stage liver disease caused by alcoholism. She has been sober for 12 months, yet her liver is too damaged to recover. The only treatment option for Barbara is a liver transplant, but the waiting list for a donor organ from a deceased person in the area where she lives is six months and she is unlikely to survive that long without a new organ. Barbara's daughter, Tiffany, is 18 years old and currently unemployed. She has contacted her mother's doctor to ask if he would consider her to participate as a live organ donor for her mother. The doctor talks to the transplant surgeon, who suggests that an ethics consultation might be useful in determining what is best in this situation.

All across the United States there is a severe shortage of deceased donor organs. At the end of 2007 there were nearly 100,000 people needing organ transplants in the United States. These people are awaiting livers, kidneys, lungs, hearts, intestines, and pancreas tissue to be donated by others upon their death. Unlike many countries in Europe, where the law presumes that people would agree to donate after death unless they voice an opinion otherwise, in the United States the reverse concept operates. Specifically, it is presumed that individuals do *not* want to donate their organs unless they have voiced their consent to donate by registering such (at their motor vehicle department, for example) or telling their family. Few people chose to register as organ donors.

While some people have personal or philosophical reasons for choosing not to be organ donors, there are many myths about organ donation and transplantation that underlie some decisions not to register. For example, some people believe that registering to donate will result in less medical treatment being provided them when they are critically ill, so that they will die quickly (making their organs available). Some believe that if their organs are removed their bodies won't be suitable for an open casket funeral. Some believe that transplantation is experimental technology and that their family will be charged for the organ donation surgery. In some cultures, it is believed that removal of organs compromises one's future life. Sale of the donated organs for profit is also another fear, as is unfair allocation of the organ (e.g., the hospital might selectively give the organ to a wealthy person instead of the person who clinically needs it the most, regardless of their financial, racial, or social status). These are myths.

In the United States, deceased donor organs are allocated according to a system (called a protocol) defined by the United Network for Organ Sharing (UNOS; www.unos.org). These protocols are designed only to consider clinically relevant features. Thus, they take account of clinical need (how sick the patient is) and the length of time the patient has been waiting for a transplant, as well as other factors such as organ size and blood type of the donor and recipient. Wealth, social status, occupation, religion, and race are all rigorously excluded from these protocols. A national computerized database is maintained by UNOS to track all those waiting for and receiving donor organs.

Because there is such a drastic shortage of deceased donor organs available, new approaches have developed so that transplants of all major organs except the heart may occur through a process known as "live donation." In live donation, a healthy adult gives a kidney, lung lobe, intestinal segment, liver tissue, or pancreas tissue while he or she is alive to a patient in need of transplant. These organs, or parts of organs, can be removed without serious damage, although at some risk to the donor. In the case of live lung donation, two live donors each donate one lung lobe for placement into one patient. In the case of live liver donation, liver tissue (segment or lobe) is removed from the donor and given to the patient. The remaining liver tissue in the donor will grow, returning the liver to its original size within 4–6 weeks.

Living donation is not without risk to the donor. In fact there have been several deaths of live liver and kidney donors around the world. The risk of surgical complications, including death, is one reason that the informed consent process and health screening of the donors are very important. To this end, in the United States, federal regulations require that a donor advocate or donor advocate team assist donor candidates with questions about safety or ethics throughout the screening and post-donation periods. This person/group is separate from the team that takes care of the organ recipient so that there is no conflict of interest or pressure to promote the donation if safety or ethical issues are identified.

The ethical basis of organ donation is altruism, the willingness to help another even at cost to oneself. Thus, in most countries of the world selling organs is considered unethical. In the United States, it is illegal to sell human organs. A live donor cannot sell his or her organ or tissue to the recipient, and the recipient cannot provide money to the donor as payment for the organ/tissue. Such an act is punishable with five years in federal prison and/or $50,000 in fines. The medical and surgical expenses of live donors are paid by the recipients' transplant insurance, but live donors usually do incur costs that are considered out-of-pocket expenses (e.g., lost time from work, childcare expenses). Because of this, donor candidates need to assure themselves and the advocate/advocate team that they can afford to participate. Donors must not ask their organ recipients for money or other forms of payment (e.g., employment, car, vacations) before or after donation. These contaminate the altruistic foundation of live donation and create conflict of interest on the part of the donor.

Whether the organ is from a live or deceased donor, the organ is a gift that must be cherished by the recipient. Transplant patients have an ethical duty to be "good stewards" of the organs that are given to them. Specifically, this entails ensuring that everything that fosters the health of the organ must be a priority in the patient's life. Activities and behaviors that promote organ health include taking anti-rejection medication as prescribed, not using tobacco or illicit drugs, maintaining a healthy weight, keeping physically fit, and attending all scheduled medical appointments. For those who have received a new liver, alcohol abstinence is essential.

As shown, the duties required of organ stewardship are many. For some patients, these duties are too rigorous and the medical team concludes it would be ethically inappropriate for them to receive an organ transplant because the transplant has a high likelihood of failing. Often these patients have a history of non-compliance, such as failing to take their medications as prescribed, frequently missing or canceling their medical appointments, and continuing to use alcohol, tobacco, or illicit drugs although told to stop. Some patients resist taking direction from the medical team and are unable to establish a therapeutic alliance with the physicians. In these situations, the patient is often considered too high risk for transplantation, as the team fears the patient will not take care of and respect a donated organ. These considerations may appear to be prejudicial to certain types of persons, for example, alcoholics or persons with high-risk life-styles (e.g., incarcerated). Yet they truly belong to the medical aspects relevant to the transplant decision. Both medical and psychosocial issues can affect transplant outcomes, so they are considered by a "transplant selection committee" rather than one physician. These committees consist of physicians, surgeons, nurses, social workers, psychologists, ethicists, and dieticians who review the clinical and psychosocial details of patients needing transplantation. Patients can be declined for medical reasons (they are too sick or not sick enough) and/or psychosocial reasons (noncompliant, unmotivated, suicidal).

Scientists continue to explore the concept of implanting animal organs into humans (xenotransplantation) as another possible way to alleviate the organ shortfall. The most famous xenotransplant occurred at California's Loma Linda University Medical Center in 1984. Using an experimental protocol approved by the facility's research review committee (institutional review board) 14-day-old "Baby Fae," who was born with a severely underdeveloped heart, received the walnut-sized heart of a baboon that had been raised especially for the procedure. The infant survived for 20 days but died from heart failure caused by her body rejecting the animal organ.

There are many concerns about xenotransplantation. Some concerns involve safety: will animal organs transmit new or untreatable diseases to humans? Other concerns focus on ethics. Some argue that placing animal parts into human bodies is morally wrong; however, doctors already do this on a daily basis. Some skin grafts and heart valves are harvested from pigs, for example. Others argue that animals should not be used for transplant because the action is such that humans take over the lives of the animals and use them for their own purposes, without regard for the fact that the animal dies as a result of donating (and the animal cannot consent/refuse to participate). Another issue that troubles some is that it seems that, for xenotransplantation to be successful, animals will have to be genetically modified so that their organs will not be viewed as "foreign" and rejected by the human body. This genetic manipulation of animals is seen by some as unethical because the animals, in their natural state, are healthy and need no genetic alteration. The "enhancement" is strictly for human benefit. There is no benefit to the animal, and there may, in fact, be harms (e.g., unsafe genetic defects) as the animal matures.

In the case example, while Tiffany is only 18 years old, she is a legal adult, and as an adult she is allowed to make her own medical decisions. This said, she should be allowed to present herself to the donor advocate team for evaluation as a live donor. Medical, surgical, ethical, and psychosocial evaluations will determine if she is a suitable candidate to donate a portion of her liver to her mother. The ethical concerns that will be addressed include: *Does Tiffany, while an adult, understand the donation procedure and its risks? Is Tiffany prepared for the potential financial implications of being a living donor (e.g., some uncompensated medical expenses, inability to work/interview for jobs during surgical recovery)?* The transplant team should also counsel Barbara (the mother) that she can seek a transplant evaluation at another hospital. While the waiting list in the area where she lives is six months, in some areas of the United States the waiting time for a liver is much shorter and sometimes patients move temporarily in order to be wait listed at a transplant center with shorter waiting times.

Key Points

- *Worldwide, the number of donated organs does not meet the demand.*

- *Transplantation is not an experimental technology but rather standard of care for patients with end-stage organ failure.*

- *Organs are allocated to patients based on their capacity to benefit from them, not according to their personal financial worth, social status, or moral character.*

- *Living donation is a beneficial technology, but donors must be healthy and be able to provide informed consent without coercion or conflict of interest.*

- *In the United States, a donor advocate or donor advocate team is available to assist donor candidates with questions about safety or ethics throughout the screening and post-donation periods.*

- *Patients who receive organ transplants have an ethical duty to take care of the organ so as to respect the donated gift of life.*

12

NEUROETHICS

Adam is 52 years old and has severe Parkinson's disease. His wife, Ellen, is his full-time caretaker, driving him to all his medical appointments and even assisting him with eating because his arms shake so severely. Although he is receiving medical treatment to alleviate the symptoms of Parkinson's disease, Adam remains profoundly depressed, has severe balance problems, low-volume muffled speech, and significant tremors. Adam is mentally intact and is able to make his own medical decisions. Adam and Ellen are considering a treatment they saw advertised on television, deep brain stimulation (DBS). DBS therapy is approved for the treatment of Parkinson's disease by the U.S. Food and Drug Administration. This treatment involves a surgical procedure in which a device called a neurostimulator is implanted under the skin in the chest with wires that travel up the neck and into the brain. These wires deliver electrical stimulation to targeted areas in the brain, blocking the abnormal nerve signals that cause tremors and other symptoms. The symptom that Adam most hopes to have controlled is *his low-volume muffled speech because this causes him to have feelings of anxiety and suffocation. Adam wants to regain clear, loud speech. His doctor tells him that there is no guarantee that DBS will have any effect on his speech problem. The doctor does believe, however, that this treatment will significantly reduce Adam's tremors so that he could likely feed himself.*

The brain is the body's multi-tasking organ. Not only is it the center of perception and cognition, with its vast network of cells involved in vision, movement, and thinking, but it is also the center of stimulation that keeps the heart beating and lungs breathing. It is not surprising then that, when illness affects the brain, many symptoms can emerge. For example, amyotrophic lateral sclerosis (ALS or Lou Gehrig's disease) is a disease of the nerve cells in the brain and spinal cord that are responsible for voluntary muscle movement. People with ALS have nerve cells that stop working, meaning that the brain can no longer tell the muscles to move. When the chest muscles can no longer move, ALS patients require artificial respiration. Epilepsy is a brain disorder in which abnormal electrical activity in the brain causes abnormal movements (seizures) and even loss of consciousness in some people. Many people with epilepsy cannot safely drive cars, mountain climb, or SCUBA dive.

While many symptoms of brain disorders can be treated with medication, many others cannot—and the untreated symptoms can be debilitating. This can severely impact a person's quality of life. The idea of surgical treatment of the brain raises many ethical issues. As stated, the brain is the source of control for breathing and heart function. Damage to the areas of the brain that control these functions can be fatal. The brain is also the core of one's personality and emotions. Certain types of brain damage can change one's personality. For example, some people with damage in the fronto-temporo-limbic regions display addictive behaviors such as pathologic (excessive and harmful) gambling. The brain is also the source of our ability to think and process information. When significant brain damage occurs, our ability to function in daily life and make decisions for ourselves can be severely impaired. Surgically treating the brain is delicate work that often cannot be reversed if there is a mistake.

Many brain surgeries involve removing portions of the brain. Sometimes, even half the brain is removed. This is called a hemispherectomy, and is usually performed in cases of severe, uncontrolled epilepsy. When portions of the brain are removed, they do not grow back. If healthy brain tissue is removed, it is gone forever. When a diseased portion of the brain is removed, there is always a risk that a person will lose normal functioning that the removed or adjacent areas of the brain may have provided. For example, surgery on areas of the brain that control speech and language has the risk of leaving the patient with speech difficulties (e.g., stuttering, mumbling, cannot think of the "right" word). Other forms of brain surgery include stimulating the brain with electricity (as in Adam's case) and deadening a portion of the brain so that it is no longer active. In addition to the risks already mentioned, brain surgery can also result in bleeding, infection, memory loss, and stroke.

Because the symptoms of brain and neurological disease can be devastating, patients and families are faced with tough choices when their doctors offer surgical therapies. Patients and families should have realistic expectations with regard to surgical outcomes. Surgical risks can be significant and permanent. Not pursuing surgery and remaining burdened with symptoms is also significant. Further, sometimes these symptoms become progressive or permanent. Weighing the risks and benefits of surgery versus medical therapy must be carefully done by physicians, patients, and families; often, this involves serious ethical consideration to ensure the patient is making an informed choice.

A coma is a complex neurological phenomenon that can be caused by a variety of events, including direct damage to the brain by a head injury, infection, or poisoning with chemicals, drugs, or alcohol. When a patient is comatose, the brain is affected in such a way that the patient cannot be aroused to consciousness, cannot communicate, and cannot move voluntarily. When a coma lasts at least 30 days it is termed a persistent vegetative state (PVS). During the first few days of a coma, it is sometimes difficult for doctors to determine the patient's prognosis—that is, whether there is a chance that the coma will end and the patient will return to consciousness. It can also be difficult to determine what level of function the patient will have: Will he or she be able to walk? Talk? Make complex decisions?

When a neurologist makes a diagnosis of PVS, he or she is quite certain that the patient's level of functioning will not improve from that noted at the time of diagnosis. PVS patients are bed-bound and rely on a feeding tube and often a ventilator to survive. These patients cannot speak or respond to verbal instructions, and they cannot perform routine hygiene activities such as bathing or oral care. When surrogates are faced with either a coma or PVS diagnosis, medical teams often initiate discussions about quality of life and patient values. If various technological treatments, such as respirators or dialysis, are keeping the patient alive but not giving a life of quality that is consistent with the patient's values and wishes, surrogates need to discuss this with the medical team. It is important that surrogates and physicians provide treatment that benefits the patient and honors the values and wishes of the patient. However, in PVS, it can be argued that the patient, who has no consciousness or experience, has no quality of life and that no human would wish to live in this way. The general, although not universal, opinion of bioethicists is that patients for whom a definite diagnosis of PVS has been made may be allowed to die. U.S. law has generally supported this opinion; however, every case must be thoughtfully considered, and an ethics consultation can sometimes be helpful to families and surrogates who find themselves in these complex situations.

In the case example, it is clear that the treatment that the doctor is offering will not satisfy the expectations of the patient. This is an important fact to know, because the DBS is an invasive surgery that should not be employed in situations of unrealistic benefit. The neurologist might consider offering other potential therapies that specifically address Adam's speech defect, because this is what is most important to the patient. If this deficit can be combated, the patient might be more receptive to addressing his other symptoms as well.

KEY POINTS

- *When significant brain damage occurs, our ability to function in daily life and make decisions for ourselves can be severely impaired.*

- *The brain is the core of one's personality and emotions.*

- *Surgical treatment of the brain raises ethical issues.*

- *Brain surgery has risks that are significant and permanent.*

- *PVS is a permanent state of unconsciousness in which patients cannot make voluntary movements or communicate and they rely on others for all their daily needs.*

13

ETHICS AND
REPRODUCTIVE
TECHNOLOGY

A nn and Abe have been married for five years. They have *been trying to conceive a child for the past two years. Both underwent thorough infertility testing, and it was concluded that Ann cannot bear children because she has a malformed uterus. The couple decided to create a set of embryos using Abe's sperm and Ann's eggs. Ann's doctor implanted three embryos into the womb of Ann's sister, Cindy, who agreed to be a surrogate mother. The procedure was successful, and Ann and Abe have been paying for all of Cindy's prenatal care as well as giving her $50 a week for food. During the sixth month of pregnancy, Cindy asked Ann and Abe to buy her a new car. Feeling stressed and afraid, Ann and Abe informed the doctor of the surrogate's request. The doctor arranged for a "surprise" meeting of everyone involved at Cindy's next check-up, and included the ethicist associated with the clinic.*

Reproductive medicine is ethically interesting for many reasons, principally because it technologically enhances or replaces the form of reproduction practiced by humans since time immemorial. However, it is also interesting because it is not a treatment necessary for *preservation* of any patient's life. Many dilemmas that occur in hospitals and health care involve decisions about allowing a patient to die or preserving a life that is badly damaged. Reproductive medicine is unique (and optional) because childbirth and fathering children are not essential to saving one's own life. These activities are indeed frequently deeply desired and life enhancing, but they lack the medical necessity associated with life saving. Only in one respect can reproductive technologies be likened to other medical treatments: when it corrects a physical defect in a person's reproductive capacity, such as blocked ovaries or inability to produce sperm.

Assisted reproduction is also ethically complex because it focuses so directly on very complex notions: "personhood"—determining when life begins—and "parenthood"—who counts as parents when multiple parties contribute to conception and pregnancy. The concept of personhood is very complex; there are many theories about when an embryo or fetus is considered a person. Some of these theories appeal to science, others to law, while still others appeal to religion. At one end of the spectrum, there are opinions that argue that an embryo (a successfully fertilized egg that has begun cell division but is not more than eight weeks old) should be designated a person. At the other end of the spectrum, there are opinions that argue that a fetus is not a person until it leaves the womb at birth. In between, there are many, many theories. All of these theories are open to debate, because there is no definitive proof for any of them. As an example of this confusion, the most famous legal case about abortion, *Roe v. Wade*, went before the United States Supreme Court. Opposing sides constructed their arguments around two quite different theories—the legal view that personhood begins at birth, and the philosophical-medical view that a fetus mature enough to be born live might be treated as if it is a person.

Parenthood is another difficult concept, made even more difficult due to the many assisted-reproduction technologies available. "Conventional" parenthood is generally understood as a couple that generates and raises a child. Also, adults who adopt live children are considered "parents." However, reproductive technologies provide many variations on these arrangements. Surrogate mothers add a new person to the family picture. A surrogate mother carries and births the child who has been conceived with sperm and egg of other persons and then surrenders the child to the woman who requested the surrogacy. Usually, the surrogate mother provides the egg, but sometimes the surrogate requester provides her own eggs for the procedure. Additionally, a child birthed by a surrogate mother can be conceived using donor sperm or sperm from the partner of the surrogacy requester. Surrogacy in its smallest form creates a triad family (surrogate birth mother, persons requesting surrogacy and also providing sperm and egg). Surrogacy in its largest form creates a family of five (surrogate birth mother, persons requesting surrogacy, and the sperm and egg donors). Sometimes it is a single person, rather than a couple, who seeks a surrogate birth mother. Another variation is embryo adoption. In these situations, a person or couple adopts a frozen embryo that was created by the egg and sperm of two other people. The embryo is transferred to the womb of the adopting mother or to a surrogate mother.

In all of these configurations, concerns about surrogacy generally focus on the possibility that the surrogate will not surrender the child to the requesting individual/couple. Also, for the nine months of pregnancy, the prospective family relies on the surrogate mother to nurture the fetus appropriately. Problems of either sort can cause significant turmoil and stress. As in the case described, there is a risk that the surrogate mother could make financial demands on the prospective parents, essentially bartering for the child. It is advised that surrogacy arrangements be described in a formal contract. Consultation with an attorney familiar with these issues is recommended. Of note, the Roman Catholic Church does not accept surrogacy because it is contrary to the unity of marriage (it brings a third person, or more, into a marriage). Islam also forbids surrogacy, but Judaism and Buddhism do not.

Some women utilize either artificial insemination or in vitro fertilization (IVF) when they lack a sexually potent male partner but are able to bear a child themselves. In the simplest procedure, artificial insemination, sperm from a donor is injected into the uterus. During IVF, the woman's eggs are removed and fertilized outside her body by donor sperm. The resulting zygote is then placed in the woman's uterus for implantation. In both of these scenarios, surrogacy is avoided and thus the issue of motherhood goes without question. There are forms of IVF that do use donor eggs. When this occurs, a new variable to the parenthood concept is added. Usually, whenever donor eggs and donor sperm are used for assisted reproductive technologies, the identity of the donor remains confidential. Only under unique or predefined circumstances will the donor's identity be released to the receiving parents and resultant child. This is to protect the privacy of the donor and his or her family.

IVF frequently results in the birth of twins or even triplets. When fertilized eggs are placed into the uterus, it has been common to insert several, because implantation of the egg in the womb is not inevitable. Sometimes, however, several inserted eggs do implant, and each can begin to develop into an independent fetus. The gestation of twins or triplets (or more) is dangerous to each fetus, and sometimes to the mother. Multiple births often produce babies who are premature and in need of intensive medical treatments to survive. Sometimes, doctors advise "reducing" one fetus—that is, causing its death in the womb—yet this medical intervention poses an ethical dilemma for many. It can be an agonizing decision for those who have gone to great lengths to become parents. It is equivalent to an abortion, which many couples consider immoral. It may also be repugnant to the physician.

The financial compensation of those who donate sperm and eggs has been the subject of much ethical discussion. Sperm donors run very little risk, and, because sperm are created on a daily basis, they have an ongoing supply. These donors usually receive about $50 per donation. Egg donors, on the other hand, expose themselves to numerous and significant medical risks. In a normal menstrual cycle, one egg matures and, at ovulation, is released. In egg donation, the goal is to obtain several mature eggs. To do this, a woman's ovaries must be stimulated by high doses of injected hormones ("controlled hyperstimulation"). These hormones are injected either under the skin or into a muscle and can cause a condition called ovarian hyperstimulation syndrome (OHSS): fluid retention and swelling of the ovaries that can cause abdominal pain, pressure, swelling, blood clots, kidney failure, fluid build-up in the lungs, and shock. In rare cases, one or both ovaries must be surgically removed. Death has also occurred. Because of these significant risks, and the pain and duration of the procedure, egg donors generally receive several thousand dollars for their participation.

Some have argued that only married, heterosexual couples should have access to assisted reproduction technologies. While these arguments frequently arise from religious teachings about procreation and parenting, they are sometimes based on philosophical claims about the natural and moral desirability of dual and, usually, heterosexual parenthood for the welfare of the child. These views are, however, disputed by many sociological and psychological studies that detect no significant risks to children. There is no evidence that children raised by single parents or by gays and lesbians are harmed or disadvantaged by that fact alone.

Referring back to the case example, a family meeting was held with Cindy, Ann, Abe, the obstetrician, and the clinic's ethicist. Cindy was informed that extortion is unethical. Also, the surrogacy contract that Cindy, Abe, and Ann had signed was presented and discussed at this meeting by the ethicist, and the obstetrician formally recorded meeting minutes. The extensive conversation identified that Cindy was having transportation troubles that were causing her to have difficulty in getting to her prenatal visits. Cindy was advised that this situation did not require Ann and Abe to buy her a new car. Offering to help, the obstetrician agreed to provide Cindy with free taxi vouchers for her remaining pre-natal and post-operative clinic visits. Cindy was advised by the ethicist that, if she persists in her request for a new car (or other non-essential items), local law enforcement would be notified.

Key Points

- *Assisted reproductive technologies are ethically complex because of issues such as personhood and parenthood.*

- *There are no federal or state laws specifically governing the adoption of embryos, though some states do have laws generally related to embryo donation and or assisted-reproductive technology.*

- *There are no grounds in medicine or social science to deny assisted-reproductive technologies to single people or homosexual couples who evidence the desire and capacity to be suitable parents. However, many offer religious and ethical arguments against these arrangements.*

- *Sperm donation is a very low-risk procedure; however, egg donation is a high-risk procedure that has many potential complications, including death.*

14

GENETICS AND ETHICS

Georgette, a 20-year-old college student, recently partici-
pated in a research study and found out that she has
the gene associated with Huntington's disease, which
causes degeneration of nerve cells leading to loss of movement
control as well as mental impairment. Symptoms usually appear
between ages 30 and 40 years, and there is no cure. Georgette
shows no symptoms of the disease (and she might never, depending on several genetic factors). She is engaged to her high school
sweetheart, Ted, and their extravagant wedding is just three
months away. Georgette knows that she has a 50-50 chance of
having a child that will develop Huntington's disease. She won-
ders if she should tell Ted about her genetic status? She fears Ted
might cancel the wedding.

Genes are segments of a large molecule called DNA (deoxyribonucleic acid) that resides in almost every cell of the body.
Genes direct the formation of substances that produce the
forms and functions of the body, and they are inherited in

certain patterns. Genes influence our bodily appearance and organic functions as well as our character and behavior. Genes also influence our susceptibility to diseases such as cancer and atherosclerosis. In recent years, tremendous advances have allowed science to identify genes and their defects and link them to personal health and characteristics. There are many ethical issues associated with the topic of genetics. Knowing the patient's genetic composition might help doctors find a way to correct a defective gene or to treat a disease condition that is caused by the defect. At the present time, attempts to correct defective genes are still highly experimental. A number of diseases can be linked to defective genes, but this information usually leads to preventive efforts rather than cure. For example, a certain rare gene defect shows a high risk of developing breast or ovarian cancer; preventive medicine consists of surgical removal of the breasts and ovaries before cancer develops. Often, gene defects that can be identified are associated with diseases for which there are no known treatments, and the patient is left with information that does not personally help and, in fact, could be harmful. As an example, there is a test that can reveal a remote possibility that a person will develop Alzheimer's disease: a person informed of that risk may live for years with a worry that will never become a reality. On the other hand, early signs of Alzheimer's will be quickly recognized and preparations for a life of declining mental capacity can be made.

It is essential to recognize three facts about genetic testing. First, tests, with a few exceptions, do not predict disease. Rather, they reveal a statistical possibility, not an assurance, that a future disease might develop. Second, even when genetic information suggests increased risk of a disease, it rarely predicts the severity of that disease. Third, genetic tests that aim to determine personality and behavioral characteristics (and, to some extent, physical appearance) uncover only one contribution to these features. This is because nurturing, training, and social influences also contribute. Genetic testing very rarely provides a simple yes or no answer about disease possibility and seriousness. Also, all genetic tests require the expert interpretation of a professional. Thus, a patient who faces genetic testing must have a very clear understanding about what the test is for and how reliable it is.

Genetic information can be misused with significant negative consequences; thus, people need to be protected. In 2008, the U.S. Congress passed the Genetic Information Nondiscrimination Act (GINA). This legislation prohibits insurance companies from discrimination by reducing coverage or increasing premiums, and prohibits employers from making adverse employment decisions based on knowledge of a person's genetic code. Insurers and employers are not allowed to request or demand genetic tests. The majority of states in the United States also have safeguards for genetic information that exceed the protections provided for other types of health information. State genetic privacy laws (Appendix A) typically restrict parties such as insurers or employers from using genetic procedures without consent of the patient/employee. Actions requiring consent include performing a genetic test, accessing genetic data, storing genetic data, and disclosing genetic data.

It is important that you know your rights with regard to genetic testing. When in doubt, ask questions. Don't consent to genetic testing unless you understand its purpose, risks, and benefits. Unfortunately, it is difficult to obtain clear and accurate information about genetics. Many physicians lack the specialized training in genetics to explain the details of many genetic traits and tests. There is a special profession, genetic counseling, that does this, but there are relatively few of these professionals. Frequently, the ethical implications of testing are best understood by bioethicists.

Another ethical issue in genetic testing relates to the specialty of reproductive medicine. Some parents seek testing of their embryo or fetus in order to determine if a genetic defect (or risk of future disease) is present. If there is a history of hereditary disease in the family, this is a sensible course of action. Some worry that parents will use genetic testing as a way to self-select for the perfect child (e.g., high intellect, no physical defects, no propensity for being overweight). This would result in parents aborting a fetus that did not meet their specifications. "Normal" but "undesirable" fetuses would be aborted even though the pregnancy was planned. Almost no form of genetic testing can presently provide information of this sort. Also, even when a test is available, genetic testing is not 100 percent accurate. This means that "incorrect" data would also be gathered, also potentially resulting in abortions of planned pregnancies.

In the case example, Georgette is in the midst of an ethical dilemma. A bioethicist would suggest that she and Ted go together for a consultation with a professional genetic counselor. Unless Georgette herself is willing to call off the wedding, she should not proceed with the wedding without telling her fiancé the fact that she might develop Huntington's disease, and that she has the potential to pass the gene to future children. The genetic counselor, not the bioethicist, is in the best position to explain the genetic features that contribute to Georgette, herself, experiencing Huntington's disease, the probability of progeny inheriting the disease, as well as options of birth control and assisted reproduction.

Key Points

- *Genetic testing provides information that carries significant risk of inaccuracy.*

- *Genetic testing requires expert interpretation.*

- *Genetic information can be misused with significant negative consequences; thus, people need to be protected.*

- *The majority of states in the United States have safeguards for genetic information that go beyond the protections provided for other types of health information (Appendix A).*

- *Don't consent to genetic testing unless you understand its purpose, risks, and benefits.*

15

PEDIATRIC ETHICS

Maurice and Ann are the parents of Joseph, who is 15 years old. Joseph has Down syndrome, a condition that limits the capacity for mental development in varying degrees. He is a cheerful, highly verbal young man, but is quite seriously limited in his intellectual abilities. Joseph has been hospitalized 25 times since he was born because he has multiple medical problems commonly associated with Down syndrome. Well known to the doctors and nurses, Joseph has good relationships with the teams and never refuses treatment, even when it involves needles, catheters, or surgery. Maurice and Ann have been told that Joseph has developed end-stage heart failure caused by a virus and the only cure is a heart transplant. The success of heart transplant in people with Down syndrome is very good, comparable to that of those without Down syndrome. However, Maurice and Ann believe that a heart transplant is a procedure that Joseph would not be able to handle emotionally. They worry he would be scared by the idea of having another person's heart inside his body. They prefer to take Joseph to

Mexico for a trial of "herbal therapy," and if that does not work they will pursue hospice at home. The consensus of the heart transplant team is that Joseph is an excellent medical and surgical candidate and he should be placed on the organ waiting list, as it is a life-saving opportunity. Some people on the team wonder if the parents find the transplant care needs too burdensome; others believe that the parents, although very devoted to Joseph, would be relieved if he died. The parents are threatening to take Joseph out of the hospital by force if they are not allowed to refuse this procedure. The doctors seek an ethics consultation.

Parental decision-making about their children in times of medical crisis can be very difficult. Parents are under an enormous amount of pressure, often performing multiple roles at the same time: spouse, employee, caregiver, accountant/banker, mentor, supervisor, and educator. During a medical crisis, these roles often do not end because they cannot be shifted to other people. Parents who have a very sick child are inundated with medical terms and medical personnel, and surrounded by the sometimes intimidating setting of a medical ward. They see their child suffering and they want to intervene, but they frequently are faced with numerous, difficult choices.

Overall, the role of the parent is to protect the child and to ensure that he or she obtains all needed medical care. Sometimes the medical treatment that is needed is painful or causes side effects such as hair loss, weight loss, and infection. Some treatments last for weeks or months (e.g., ventilator support, chemotherapy, artificial feeding). This often removes children from their daily activities such as school, scouts, and sports. The rigors of a child's treatment also can take parents away from their jobs and their other children. When children have had multiple hospitalizations, parents can become very stressed, as can the other, healthy children in the family. If lengthy hospitalizations and treatments are proposed, parents may wonder whether their child can tolerate them and how they will affect the child's quality of life. These situations are especially difficult when the child is young, as yet unable to form opinions and even effectively communicate his or her feelings.

In these situations, it is very important for families to work closely with the medical team and others, such as social workers and spiritual care counselors. These allies, working together, can create a care plan that reflects on both quality of life and the child's welfare. When the child is experiencing significant pain or other symptoms that are difficult to control, palliative medicine specialists can help (see Chapter 10). Also, an ethics consultation can provide guidance to the family and medical team (see Chapter 2).

Pediatricians and pediatric nurses are commonly very sensitive to the pressures experienced by parents of sick children, and work hard to alleviate the burdens, but at times disagreement might arise between parents and caregivers. In situations of impasse between parents and the medical team, the welfare of the child remains the priority—but the disagreement might be precisely about what constitutes the welfare of the child. Medical personnel may view a medical treatment in light of their experience, or may consider even partial success as worthwhile. Parents may focus on the immediate suffering that the treatment causes their child, or desire nothing but a complete cure.

Disagreement over the welfare of a child, particularly a child with severe illness, is unquestionably a disagreement over values. For some, the value of continued life itself is primary; for others, the value of *quality* of life is more highly esteemed. Bioethics issues have been involved in this debate, and have been central to dealing with many widely known cases. Thus, an ethics consultation may allow the diverse viewpoints to be aired, facts to be clarified, and options explored.

In the United States, law establishes child protective agencies to deal with irreconcilable conflicts over the welfare of children. These agencies can obtain temporary control over a child when there is evidence that a child may be harmed by the decisions or neglect of parents. Sometimes the decisions must go to a court for adjudication. The reason for this is that, in the United States, parents are not allowed to refuse standard-of-care medical treatments for their children (although in some states, religious preferences for spiritual over medical care, and religious objections to certain forms of treatment, such as immunization, may be permitted by statutory law). If a refusal can lead to serious harm, courts can order these treatments performed against the parents' wishes. Courts sometimes allow older children (teenagers) to make their own medical decisions and allow them to refuse medical care if the judge believes that the child is making an informed refusal.

In the case example, an ethics consultation would first clarify the facts of the situation, verifying the medical data and the differing positions of the contesting parties. Then, a family meeting would be held in which parents and providers could talk together. Also, it would be helpful to interview the patient in private, to attempt to learn his level of understanding of his personal situation with regard to his medical condition and the concept of heart transplantation. The views of the parents may be very valid. Consultations from additional specialists, such as those from the fields of psychology and child development, might also be sought. The patient and parents should also be given the opportunity to meet with others who have received a heart transplant to learn from their experiences directly. A second opinion would likely be helpful in this case and would give the family the sense that their concerns are being heard. Also, if they hear a medical consensus that surgery is in the patient's best interest, this may cause them to move forward with the procedure. If there is still resistance to surgery in the face of a medical consensus that such would be standard of care, the medical team could approach the legal system for a court order to allow the surgery to occur.

KEY POINTS

- *Parents have the moral duty, and usually the desire, to protect and promote the welfare of their children when illness requires treatment.*

- *Parents cannot refuse standard-of-care medical treatments for their children, if that refusal may seriously harm the child. Courts can order these treatments be performed against the parents' wishes.*

- *Courts sometimes allow older children (teenagers) to make their own medical decisions and allow them to refuse medical care if the judge believes that the child is making an informed refusal.*

16

Participating in a Research Study

John is 30 years old and works two part-time jobs, neither of which provides health insurance. Despite eating a low-fat, low-acid diet, and not being overweight, John has persistent heartburn. Sometimes the heartburn is so painful that it wakes him up at night. Last week an advertisement in the local newspaper caught John's eyes: "Is Heartburn Making Your Life Miserable? Call 1-800-HOT-STUDY." The ad stated that volunteers would not have to pay for "study medication" and they would receive $100 for participating. John called and spoke with a nurse, who explained that a group of gastroenterologists was studying an experimental heartburn drug. John decided to enroll in the study. He appeared at the office, met briefly with a nurse who explained the study, and signed a consent form. He took the experimental drug for six weeks and received two free examinations of his throat, esophagus, and stomach with an endoscope—a long tube with a camera at the tip. John also kept a diary of his daily meals and physical symptoms. Most of the time, John felt terrible, with flu-like symptoms, agitation, and nausea. He told his friend,

"That medicine is a flop! I'm no better than I was when I started, plus I feel sick all the time."

Medical research is essential for progress in medical science. Participants in research make a significant and sometimes courageous contribution to science and the welfare of others. However, few people really understand what research is and how it is carried out. Today, it is quite possible that any patient of any doctor might be invited to be a participant in research. Thus, it is important to understand what that invitation entails.

Research is not the same as standard clinical practice, but many people do not know the difference. Even though much research takes place in hospitals and doctor's offices and employs standard medical procedures such as drawing blood and collecting urine, standard medical practice aims to diagnose and treat a disease with common, accepted treatments. Research, also called experimental medicine or clinical investigation, aims to gather information that might improve scientific understanding of a particular disease and possibly be helpful to future patients—it does not aim to diagnose or treat disease for the research subjects who are enrolled in the study project. Formally, research is the practice of following a set plan, called a protocol, to collect and analyze information that develops or contributes to general scientific knowledge. In many of these protocols, participants are randomly divided between those who will receive the test drug and those who will receive a dummy drug, called a placebo, so that they can be compared. This sort of division must be explained to the participant, but often they don't fully understand.

In the United States, research protocols involving humans must be approved by a research review committee known as an Institutional Review Board (IRB) before the study can begin. The protocols must contain detailed information about the purpose of the research, the type of people who will be enrolled as participants, the procedures they will undergo, and the risks of those procedures. The protocols must have scientific merit and be justified in terms of the benefit to society and the risks to participants. Also, the IRB requires a suitable method of informed consent for each person enrolling. This includes approving the consent form to ensure it accurately reflects the nature of the study, its risks and benefits, and who to contact in case of an emergency, among other items. The researcher is responsible for explaining the study to the prospective subject and asking for the subject's consent.

The data collected during research studies is for the benefit of science and future patients, not usually the research subjects currently enrolled in the experiment. Research subjects often do not understand this point and assume they will personally reap clinical benefit from participating. This misunderstanding is known as a "therapeutic misconception." In the study described above, John believed he was getting free treatment for his heartburn. This was the reason that he enrolled in the project. Ethically speaking, John's expectation of benefit from study participation was unrealistic, but it is easy to see that John is part of a vulnerable population. John is vulnerable to exploitation because he is sick and desires treatment but has no health insurance. Research teams must strive to educate potential research subjects that participation in research is not the same as health care. This is important so that subjects do not have false hopes about study participation. Also, this is important because, in the United States, there is no legal obligation for research facilities or research study sponsors to provide free medical care to research subjects who are injured or suffer clinical complications as a result of participating in a research study. These medical costs, as well as loss of income due to time away from work, can be financially significant.

Even people who are healthy and have health insurance can be vulnerable to unethical study recruitment. It is for this reason that IRBs do not allow research subjects to be recruited with promises of extravagant compensation (inappropriately large sums of money). Extravagant compensation could cause individuals to undervalue or disregard the risks of study participation, putting themselves in harm's way without serious reflection. For example, in Phase I studies, protocols do not aim to treat any disease or symptom and only healthy individuals are enrolled. Drugs are tested at escalating doses to find out how safe they are. At each dosing, the research subjects are checked to determine if they are experiencing any new symptoms, or if the symptoms they had at the lower doses increase as the amount of drug they receive increases. By studying drugs this way, researchers can determine a safe dose to start at when, in the future, they test the drug on a larger sample of people who have the disease/illness they are aiming to treat. Phase I studies have no possible therapeutic benefit, and they can expose healthy people to toxic drugs with significant side effects, so people contemplating enrolling in these studies need protections to ensure they are not being coerced with extravagant incentives to enroll.

If an experimental drug is found to be safe during Phase I study, then researchers will proceed to Phase II testing. In Phase II research studies, the experimental drug is administered to people who have the disease/illness the drug is intended to treat. A small group of sick people are enrolled, and researchers observe and test them to explore the side effects of the drug in this small population of people. The researchers will also collect preliminary data on the effectiveness of the drug on this group. If the drug successfully passes Phase II, researchers will proceed with Phase III research studies. During Phase III, the drug is tested on several hundred to several thousand people who have the disease/illness the drug is intended to treat. This allows researchers to gather a large pool of data from a large cross-section of people who have various characteristics (age, gender, race, body size, etc.). After a drug successfully completes this testing, it can be approved by the U.S. Food and Drug Administration and can be prescribed by U.S. physicians for patient care. Often, when a new drug is released, researchers continue to monitor the drug for side effects that patients may experience during routine clinical use. This is called Phase IV surveillance.

Being a research subject is praiseworthy, but there is no ethical obligation to enroll. Research participation is a completely voluntary endeavor, and subjects are allowed to stop participating even after they have started. Sometimes, however, a safe stopping point must be identified by the research team, because abruptly stopping a drug may have bad effects. Leaving a study before it is completed should not result in any personal penalties, though research subjects usually cannot expect to collect full compensation but rather prorated compensation. Because study participation is not meant to be a form of employment, compensation received reflects only the burdens placed on the research subject during participation (e.g., time commitment, parking, customary pain and suffering).

Most of the research approved in the United States is safe: it is carried out by qualified investigators, and careful attention is paid to procedures and to impact on patients. Still, research involves medical interventions that carry risks, and a small number of persons have died as a result of research participation. The research review processes established by the IRB require that all information about these matters be clearly explained, so that volunteers understand that they are entering a worthy but risky activity. Anyone invited to be a research participant should ask whether the project has passed review and should study carefully the informed consent document that he or she is required to sign.

Sometimes researchers use blood, urine, and tissue samples in their research. Often, they plan to do future research on the topic that is currently under study, and it is helpful if they have ongoing access to the samples from the primary (current) study. Usually, in order for researchers to use these primary samples for future research, they need permission from the research subject. The only time such permission is not needed is when the samples are to be stored in such a way that there is no information that links the sample to the research subject (no name, identification number, birth date, etc.). These are known as anonymous samples. Because the samples are anonymous, there are no concerns about privacy or confidentiality about the person who provided the sample. If, however, there is a way to track the sample to the identity of the research subject, then the research subject must give consent for the sample to be saved.

When research teams ask your consent to save samples, they will give you the option of consenting to general use of your sample (for research that does not involves genetics) or genetic research with your sample. As discussed in Chapter 14, genetic testing is complex and there are more risks to this type of research if the sample can be traced back to your identity. The decision is yours to make. You cannot be forced to allow your samples to be saved if you don't want them to be saved. When you refuse to give consent for your samples to be saved after the study is completed, they will be destroyed by the research team.

KEY POINTS

- *A research study is a scientific analysis to determine the effects of drugs, devices, or procedures and whether one form of treatment is safe and is superior to, or equivalent to, another.*

- *Research studies must be approved by Institutional Review Boards, and all participants must freely volunteer.*

- *Some people enroll in research studies with the hope of getting free medical care.*

- *Research studies are not designed for the therapeutic benefit of the research subject, but rather they are designed to collect information for the benefit of future patients.*

- *Potential research subjects should carefully consider the risks of study participation.*

- *Potential research subjects should read the consent form and understand it before signing it. For high-risk studies, talk to other research subjects (if possible) before agreeing to participate.*

- *There is no ethical duty or other requirement to participate in a research study. Participation is voluntary, and you may quit at any time without any penalty.*

Appendix A:
Resource List

American Medical Association. 2009. Code of Medical Ethics: Current Opinions with Annotations. Chicago: AMA. Available at: http://www.ama-assn.org/ama/pub/physician-resources/medical-ethics/code-medical-ethics.shtml.

Jonsen, A. R. 2005. *Bioethics beyond the Headlines: Who Lives? Who Dies? Who Decides?* Lanham, Md.: Rowman & Littlefield.

Jonsen, A. R, M. Siegler, and W. J. Winslade. 2006. *Clinical Ethics: A Practical Approach to Ethical Decisions in Clinical Medicine*, 6th ed. New York: McGraw-Hill.

National Commission for the Protection of Human Subjects of Biomedical and Behavioral Research. 1979. The Belmont Report: Ethical Principles and Guidelines for the Protection of Human Subjects of Research. Washington, D.C.: U.S. Department of Health and Human Services. Available at: http://www.hhs.gov/ohrp/humansubjects/guidance/belmont.htm.

National Conference of State Legislatures. 2008. Genetic Privacy Laws. Denver: NCSL. Available at: http://www.ncsl.org/programs/health/genetics/prt.htm.

New York State Task Force on Life and the Law. 2009. Thinking of Becoming an Egg Donor? Get the Facts Before You Decide! Albany: State of New York, Department of Health. Available at: http://www.health.state.ny.us/community/reproductive_health/infertility/docs/1127.pdf.

U.S. Department of Health and Human Services. Summary of the HIPAA Privacy Rule Washington, D.C.: HHS. Available at: http://www.hhs.gov/ocr/privacysummary.pdf.

U.S. National Library of Medicine. 2010. Medline Plus Medical Encyclopedia. Bethesda, Md.: NLM. Available at: http://www.nlm.nih.gov/medlineplus/encyclopedia.html.

WEB SITES:

American Society for Bioethics and Humanities (ASBH)
http://www.asbh.org

American Society for Reproductive Medicine (ASRM)
http://www.asrm.org

AskTheEthicist.com
http://www.AskTheEthicist.com

Caring Connections (advance directive templates, U.S. state-specific)
http://www.caringinfo.org/stateaddownload

Children of God for Life (advance directive template, Catholic)
http://www.cogforlife.org/Catholiclivingwill.htm

Children's Hospice and Palliative Care Coalition
http://www.childrenshospice.org

Hospice (general hospice information)
http://www.hospicenet.org

Jewish Medical Directives for Health Care (advance directive
    template, Jewish)
    http://www.rabbinicalassembly.org/docs/
    medical%20directives.pdf
Office of Research Integrity (ORI)
    http://ori.dhhs.gov
PubMed (journal article database)
    http://www.ncbi.nlm.nih.gov/sites/entrez
TransplantEthics.com
    http://www.TransplantEthics.com
United Network for Organ Sharing (UNOS)
    http://www.unos.org
U.S. Food and Drug Administration (FDA)
    http://www.fda.gov

APPENDIX B: GLOSSARY

Advance directive: a document (also known as a living will) signed by an adult who has decision-making capacity in which that person states his or her wishes about the medical care desired during a terminal illness if he or she is no longer capable of expressing his or her wishes. These documents are intended as guidance for health care providers.

Assent: the agreement by a child or mentally impaired adult to participate in research or medical therapy. This agreement is usually expressed when the person, after an explanation suited to his or her age, does not refuse. This is distinct from "informed consent" (see below).

Attending physician: a physician who has completed residency training and assumes the role of supervising physician for the hospitalized patient.

Autonomy: the right of a person to make choices about the direction of his or her life, based on his or her own values. Respect for autonomy is the moral principle that directs persons to refrain from preventing others from making and pursuing their own values and choices, unless these pose serious risks of harm to others or to the social welfare.

Best interests: a judgment about how a particular course of action will support and advance the well-being of a person who is unable to express his or her own interests. In bioethics, a method of medical decision-making that reflects on the burdens and benefits of particular treatments and attempts to determine what a hypothetical "reasonable" person would choose, when surrogates and the medical team do not know the specific wishes and values of the patient and the patient cannot express them.

Beneficence: the ethical principle that obliges one person to act so as to promote the welfare of another person. In bioethics, the duty of the physician to seek the welfare of his or her patients.

Clinical nurse specialist (CNS): a nurse with a master's or doctoral degree who has advanced clinical training. Some of these nurses have authority to diagnose simple illnesses and to prescribe medication.

Code Blue: an emergency call when a hospitalized patient is experiencing a cardiac and/or respiratory arrest. During a Code Blue, doctors and nurses perform cardiopulmonary resuscitation (CPR) in an attempt to restore normal heart rhythms.

Coma: unconsciousness caused by injury, illness, or poisoning. The patient cannot be aroused. Coma is usually temporary but after a patient has remained in a coma for at least 30 days this is referred to as a persistent vegetative state (PVS), defined below.

Confidentiality: the duty of a second party to keep private information obtained from or about a person to whom he or she is linked in a professional relationship, or bound by a promise.

Decision-making capacity (DMC): the ability of an adult to receive information about a proposed therapy, understand how it pertains to his or her specific situation, consider this information and options for choice, and express a choice about accepting or rejecting the therapy. Medical providers and ethicists have the ability to determine whether a patient has DMC. If a patient is known to lack DMC, an appropriate person, called a surrogate, must be chosen to make decisions for that person. If the choice of a surrogate is made by judicial process, the terms "competent" and "incompetent" are used.

Defibrillator: a device that provides an electrical shock to the heart to return it to normal rhythm when it beats too fast or at an irregular pace. These can be small devices implanted in the chest for regular use by patients with known heart problems, or larger devices temporarily placed on the outside of the chest in emergency situations as the need arises.

Deoxyribonucleic acid (DNA): a large molecule in every cell of the human body (except red blood cells) on which are located the genes containing information that determines organic structure and function, and, to some extent, behavioral characteristics.

Dialysis: a medical procedure that uses a machine to remove toxins, waste, and fluids from the blood of patients who have kidney failure. It may be used on a temporary basis—for example, when kidneys are damaged by poisons or on a permanent basis, several times a week for life, when kidneys are irreversible damaged.

Do not escalate (DNE): a medical decision (order) that directs the medical team to maintain the current level of treatment for a patient and not to add additional aggressive therapies to the treatment plan.

Do not resuscitate (DNR): a medical decision (order) that directs the medical team not to revive the patient by use of the procedures of cardiopulmonary resuscitation (e.g., electric shocks, chest compressions) if the patient develops a cardiac or respiratory arrest. Such an order is given only when the patient has clearly chosen not to have cardiopulmonary resuscitation or when a patient who has lost decision-making capacity, is judged terminally ill, and the procedure is unlikely to provide benefit.

Durable power of attorney for health care: the legal authorization whereby a person designates another person to act as surrogate decision maker to make decisions on his or her behalf when he or she is no longer able to make such decisions.

Euthanasia: the active and usually unlawful killing of a patient by someone administering an overdose of drugs or poison in order to end suffering. In situations of euthanasia, the patient's disease does not cause death; instead, the drug or poison does.

Feeding tube: a tube placed in the nose, mouth, or stomach and filled with liquid nutrients for patients who cannot swallow or otherwise tolerate oral feeding.

Futility: the determination by a physician that a particular treatment will not, or is highly unlikely to, provide medical benefit to the patient and change the course of that patient's disease.

Genetic testing: laboratory tests that examine a person's DNA in an effort to find genetic markers and defects associated with disease or risk of disease.

Health Insurance Portability and Accountability Act (HIPAA): U.S. federal regulation that protects a patient's medical records from being disclosed outside his or her medical providers without patient authorization. The act also gives patients the right to inspect their own records.

Hospice: a facility or program designed to provide care and control of pain, suffering, and emotional and psychological symptoms for patients who are dying and expected to have a life expectancy of six months or less. Treatment is not directed to curing disease or preventing the forthcoming death, but rather alleviating the symptoms associated with dying. Hospice services can be provided in hospitals, in special institutions, or at home.

Informed consent: a decision whereby an adult with decision-making capacity formally accepts clinical therapy or research participation after it has been thoroughly explained to him or her. Informed consent is the ethical and legal premise for any medical or research intervention.

Informed refusal: when an adult with decision-making capacity makes an informed choice to refuse a recommended medical treatment that has been thoroughly explained to him or her.

Institutional Review Board (IRB): a committee of mixed membership (scientists and non-scientists) required by U.S. federal regulations in all institutions where research is performed to review and approve research protocols involving human subjects.

Justice: the ethical principle that directs social benefits to be fairly and equitably distributed through communities and populations, and prohibits discrimination and bias.

Life support: medical treatments such as dialysis, artificial ventilation, pressor drugs, and artificial provision of nutrients and fluids that keep seriously ill patients alive by supporting or substituting for the defects of vital organs (e.g., heart, lungs, kidneys).

Living donor: a person who donates a kidney, lung lobe, bone marrow, intestinal segment, pancreas tissue, or liver tissue while alive to a patient in need of transplantation.

Nonmaleficence: the ethical principle that directs persons to refrain from causing harm to others. In medicine, it is the duty of the doctor to carefully evaluate any risks of treatment, avoid those risks as far as possible, and allow them only when balanced by the prospect of success of that treatment.

Nurse practitioner (NP): a nurse with advanced clinical training and a master's degree who can diagnose illness and prescribe medication. In some states, NPs do not have to practice along with a physician but can have their own private practices.

Pacemaker: a small device implanted in a patient's chest that uses electricity to stimulate the heart to beat faster when the natural heart rate becomes too slow.

Palliative medicine: a subspecialty of medical practice that focuses on treating or controlling a patient's pain or other debilitating symptoms such as nausea, vomiting, agitation, shortness of breath, as well as emotional and psychological distress. A palliative medicine consultation can be particularly useful in alleviating pain and distress when a patient is dying.

Persistent vegetative state (PVS): a coma lasting 30 days or longer from which the patient is highly unlikely to recover. It does not appear that persons in this state have any consciousness or experience of internal or external events, although their eyes may open and they may make inarticulate sounds and involuntary movements.

Physician assistant (PA): a specially trained person who is licensed to provide basic medical services (e.g., the diagnosis and treatment of common illnesses, perform school physicals) usually under the supervision of a licensed physician.

Physician-assisted suicide (PAS): the act of a patient causing his or her own death (in legal terms, "committing suicide") by using medication prescribed by a physician. The drug directly causes the patient's death, not the patient's underlying disease or illness. The physician must be assured that the patient who requests the drug has decision-making capacity and is terminally ill. PAS is illegal in the United States, except in Oregon.

Pressor: a drug used to raise blood pressure.

Quality of life (QOL): the judgment made by a person, or by someone observing that person, that his or her life as a whole, or in some important aspect, is good or bad, better or worse. This judgment usually looks to whether life is independent and enjoyable, emotionally and spiritually vital, free from pain and suffering, engaged in social intercourse and community, and unburdened financially. Serious defects in such aspects of life may lead a person to judge that his or her life is of poor quality, "that life is not worth living." Judgment about quality of life is properly made by the person living it. Many persons who do have serious deficits tolerate them, and even judge that their lives are good. Still, quality of life becomes an ethical problem when others, such as relatives or physicians, must ask whether quality of life is acceptable to the person who is living it, when that person is no longer capable of self-expression. A further ethical problem concerns the relevance of quality of life judgments to important medical decisions, such as withdrawing life support.

Research: a scientific study aimed at developing new knowledge. Research uses a formal plan or protocol to collect and analyze information that develops or contributes to general knowledge that will improve medical diagnosis and treatment. The data collected is for the benefit of science and future patients, not the research subject.

Research subject (or research participant): anyone who volunteers to enroll in an experiment or research study and undergoes tests, interviews, or procedures for the benefit of science and future patients.

Resident physician: also referred to as "house staff." This is an individual who has graduated from medical school and is receiving clinical training as a physician in a hospital setting. Residents are supervised by attending physicians.

Substituted judgment: decision-making by others on behalf of the patient when the surrogate knows the patient's values, because the patient has previously expressed them to the surrogate either verbally or in writing.

Surrogate: an adult who is authorized to substitute for the patient as decision-maker when the patient is unable to make his or her own medical decisions. A surrogate is usually next of kin or has been previously appointed by the patient as the holder of a durable power of attorney, but is sometimes appointed by a court procedure. A surrogate's decisions must be based on what he or she knows of the patient's own wishes or, absent this information, on a judgment of what is in the best interest of the patient.

Therapeutic alliance: the relationship between a patient and his or her health care provider in which both are working together as a team toward improving or maintaining the health of the patient.

Therapeutic misconception: when research subjects believe that participation in a research project will provide them with personal clinical benefit.

Ventilator: a machine that supports breathing through a tube placed down the patient's throat or inserted into an incision in the neck.

ABOUT THE AUTHORS

Dr. Katrina A. Bramstedt trained at Loma Linda University, UCLA, and Monash University. Dr. Bramstedt is a private practice clinical ethicist (www.AskTheEthicist.com; www.TransplantEthics.com) formerly on the faculty of The Cleveland Clinic and the California Pacific Medical Center. She has conducted more than 800 ethics consultations and written more than 70 journal articles and book chapters. Her specialty interests include transplantation, implantable medical devices, and research ethics.

Dr. Albert holds a doctorate in Religious Studies from Yale University. In 1972, he started one of the first bioethics teaching programs in the United States at the Medical School of the University of California, San Francisco, where he was director of the Division of Medical Ethics, 1973–1987. He was chairman of the Department of Medical History and Ethics at the University of Washington School of Medicine, 1987–2000. He served on two federal commissions on bioethical problems, and is member of the Institute of Medicine. He has published books on the practice, theory, and history of bioethics. Dr. Jonsen is currently the Senior Ethics Scholar in Residence, and Co-Director of the Program in Medicine and Human Values at California Pacific Medical Center, San Francisco.